Supporting People with a Learning Disability and Autistic People in Health and Social Care

Supporting People with a Learning Disability and Autistic People in Health and Social Care

Janet Finlayson

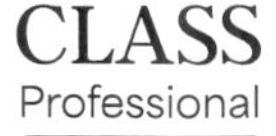

The information presented in this book is accurate and current to the best of the authors' knowledge.

The authors and publisher, however, make no guarantee as to, and assume no responsibility for, the correctness, sufficiency or completeness of such information or recommendation.

Printing history
First edition published 2025.

The authors and publisher welcome feedback from the users of this book.

Please contact the publisher:

Class Professional Publishing,
The Exchange, Express Park, Bristol Road, Bridgwater TA6 4RR
Telephone: 01278 472 800
Email: info@class.co.uk
www.classprofessional.co.uk

Class Professional Publishing is an imprint of Class Publishing Ltd
A CIP catalogue record for this book is available from the British Library

Paperback ISBN: 9781801611138
ePub ISBN: 9781801611145
ePDF ISBN: 9781801611152
Cover design by Nicky Borowiec
Designed and typeset by PHI
Printed in the UK by Hobbs

This book is printed on paper from responsible sources. Refer to local recycling guidance on disposal of this book.

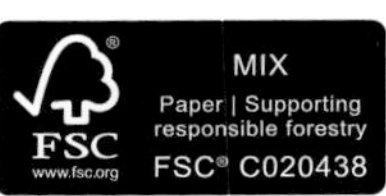

Product safety information can be found at:
https://www.classprofessional.co.uk/terms-of-use/gpsr-statement/.

Contents

Foreword

Our daughter, Laura was born with Down syndrome. She suffered severe brain damage following surgery at one year old. Laura has complex needs, but she has the nicest personality of anyone I know. We are so lucky to have her as a daughter. Every day she teaches us about what matters in life, and no matter what she is going through, she always manages a smile. Laura has two main passions in life: going out for trips in her car and 'the Singing Kettle' (a Scottish music group).

We converted an area of our house into a self-contained flat for Laura. We call it 'Laura's pad', to which she has her own front door. Laura has a personal support package and budget, which means she has her own paid support team, who provide her with support 24 hours a day, 7 days a week. This arrangement has been very successful because the support is always focused on what is best for Laura. Laura enjoys being more independent, and for us it means being her mum and dad instead of her carers. Laura is so independent now, that sometimes when I knock on the door to see how she is getting on with her support worker, she says 'bye' and shoos me out of her flat for trying to interfere or fuss over her. This makes me laugh and makes me really happy. Support that is designed around the person, according to their individual needs, works best for everyone, and should be realised for more people, as it has been for Laura and our family.

Laura has had a few negative hospital experiences, including two separate occasions of being admitted with a suspected chest infection and nearly losing her life because ward staff didn't listen to or respect us as her parents and experts who could help. These instances involved not being allowed to stay with Laura during routine procedures, medication she had been taking for over 30 years being withdrawn suddenly, not being given pain relief when it was obvious to us that she was in pain and not being allowed to follow the postural care management that we do with Laura at home. Postural care management is very important for Laura's respiratory health, as it is for other people with postural issues.

Based on Laura's and our family's experiences, I often give talks to health and social care staff at training events, seminars and conferences, so lessons can be learned from these experiences. I jumped at the chance to be part of this, to make a positive difference to the healthcare experiences of people with a learning disability and autistic people through training. I am happy to do this. But it isn't always easy for me to talk about these deeply personal matters, and at times I feel emotionally 'raw'.

This book demonstrates positive values and attitudes, and it shows throughout a respect for every individual. It's not often I come across the right values and attitudes when I am reading books about people with a learning disability and autistic people, especially if the person's disability is severe or complex. However, this book does just that while also covering so many important issues within a manageable length. The inclusion of expert voices also helps the reader to visualise the impact of these issues on real people's lives.

Marion Mcardle
Expert voice

Acknowledgements

With thanks to the expert voices for their valuable contributions. Thanks also to Brad English and Tracy Radford at OneConversation in Nottingham for their support. The expert voices are: Zahra Al Jardani, Vicky Deakin, Sam Gwynn, Shimara Hyman, Brett Kinsley, Marion Mcardle, Lizzie Quayle, Kriss Steer and Ethan Wright.

About the author

Janet Finlayson is a Registered Mental Health Nurse and Senior Research Fellow at Glasgow Caledonian University. Her research is focused on improving the health and wellbeing of people with a learning disability and autistic people. She has over thirty years' experience working with people with a learning disability, autistic people and their supporters. She also teaches research methods to postgraduate students.

People with a learning disability and autistic people

People with a learning disability and autistic people are different groups. 'People with a learning disability and autism' only refers to people with both conditions. It is respectful to refer to someone as a person with a learning disability, as you are putting the person first before their disability. However, some people, including many of the expert voices who contributed to this book, refer to themselves as being a learning-disabled person. For autistic people, some prefer the term 'people with autism', while others prefer the term 'autistic people'. The latter perceive their autism as being natural to who they are as a person; just as important to their identity as their religion, ethnicity or sexual orientation.[1] We will be referring to people with a learning disability and autistic people throughout this book, but want to stress the importance of being respectful and using the term that is preferable to the person/s to whom you are referring.

A diagnosis of 'learning disability' or 'autism' leads to better understanding of an individual's needs and helps them access appropriate health, educational and social services. Of course, a label such as 'learning disability' or 'autism' only describes part of who someone is as a person and shouldn't define them in any way that can be perceived as negative or discriminatory (for example, Petra cannot go to a music festival because she has a learning disability). People with a learning disability and autistic people are the same as everyone else, in that they are known by their names, their attributes and the meaningful relationships they have with other people. For example, my fun-loving son John or my friendly neighbour Jane.

Approximately one person in every fifty people worldwide has a learning disability, and one person in every hundred is autistic.[2]

People with a learning disability

People with a learning disability were previously defined as having all of the following three criteria:[3]

- An intelligence quotient (IQ) of less than 70
- Impairment of daily living skills
- Identification of such life-long problems before the age of 18.

According to this classification, people were described as having a mild (IQ of 50–69), moderate (IQ of 35–49), severe (IQ of 20–34) or profound (IQ below 20) learning disability. People were also defined as having a borderline learning disability (IQ of 70–85), which means having a lower than average cognitive ability.

We have come to realise over the years that defining people with a learning disability according to their IQ level is not altogether helpful, as this does not capture a person's functional level nor their ability to develop and learn. A 40-year-old man with a moderate learning disability, for example, may have an IQ level similar to that of a typical 10–11 year old (IQ 30–50), but he will also have 40 years of life experience from which he can develop and grow. The medical profession, United Kingdom (UK) governments and other relevant organisations now define people with a learning disability as having all of the following:[4,5]

- A significantly reduced ability to understand new or complex information and to learn new skills (impaired intelligence).
- A reduced ability to cope independently that started before adulthood.

There are multiple different genetic, metabolic, traumatic and infective causes of learning disability, but for many people the underlying cause is unknown. Table 1.1 provides some examples of different causes of learning disability. If you know someone with a specific learning disability condition, such as Down syndrome, it is worth learning more about the condition via trusted and reliable websites and resources, which are freely available on the internet.

Table 1.1: Examples of causes of learning disability

Causes of learning disability	Examples
Genetic	Down syndrome Fragile X syndrome Rett's syndrome
Metabolic	Phenylketonuria (PKU)
Traumatic	Birth injury (for example, interrupted oxygen supply during birth)
Infective	Measles Meningitis

The term 'learning disability' is only used and recognised in the UK. Internationally, the term is 'intellectual disability'. Both terms refer to the same group of people.

Some people with a learning disability refer to themselves as having a learning difficulty rather than a learning disability, and it is completely up to them how they wish to identify with a label that has been placed upon them. However, the term 'learning difficulty' is actually used to describe difficulties or additional support needs associated with learning, for example, dyslexia (difficulties associated with reading and spelling).[6] Understanding an individual's support needs, therefore, requires a working knowledge of what these terms accurately mean in practice.

People with a learning disability are a diverse group of people, who should be supported according to their individual needs. For example, one person with Down syndrome may live on their own and have a job, yet another person with Down syndrome may live at home with their family and require substantial support across all aspects of daily life. A person with a learning disability who is a wheelchair user will have different needs from a person with a learning disability who does not have any mobility issues but does have a visual impairment.

Autistic people

Autism is a lifelong neurodevelopmental condition that affects how a person interacts with others, communicates, learns and behaves. Autism affects how a person's brain processes information (for instance, sensory information received via sight, sound, smell, touch and taste, as well as body awareness). For example, when two people are walking through a city park and chatting, they can usually block out noises in the background and concentrate on their conversation. If one of these people is autistic, then they may not be able to block out other noises in the background (such as birds singing, park workers mowing grass with lawnmowers, dogs barking, children playing or the sound of traffic from a nearby road), and they can find this overwhelming. As another example, an autistic individual may experience the sensation of water when having a shower as hurtful 'pin pricks' on their skin, but smooth and soft surfaces may feel calming for them. These are examples only and do not apply to all autistic people, who are unique and will each experience the world in different ways.

Autism is usually known as autism spectrum disorder (ASD) because it covers a wide range (spectrum) of ways autistic people are affected by the condition, as well as a range of severity. Another term used is Autism Spectrum Condition (ASC), which is a way to acknowledge that the term 'disorder' is not helpful and can be offensive to people with the diagnosis. In general, the medical profession and other professional bodies identify autistic people as having the following characteristics:[7]

- Difficulty communicating and interacting with other people
- Restricted interests and repetitive behaviours
- Symptoms that affect their ability to function in school, work and other areas of life.

Autistic individuals may also have particular strengths or talents. These can include being able to learn things in detail and remember information for long periods of time, being strong visual and auditory learners, and excelling in maths, science, music or art.

No one knows what causes autism. However, some factors have been identified that may increase the likelihood of someone being born with autism. These factors are:[8]

- Having a brother or sister with autism
- Having older parents
- Having certain genetic conditions (for example, Down syndrome or Fragile X syndrome)
- Having a very low birth weight.

Autism, like learning disability, is not a mental illness, and autism is not associated with having had any vaccine.

Autism is a wide spectrum, and for some people the challenges they face are not as a result of their autism; they perceive their condition as being different from neurotypical people, and being different for them is part of their identity and not something that needs to be 'fixed'. The challenges they face are the expectations placed upon them by society to conform and fit in as everyone else does. For example, people with individual ways of communicating, or who cannot verbalise using words, can face a world that doesn't understand them, resulting in them being marginalised and left out of society.

It is important to know that autistic people are recognised as having a neurodivergent condition.[9,10] Neurodivergence recognises, appreciates and champions people whose brains work differently from a typical person, as everyone's brains are unique. Autistic people do experience the world we live in differently from neurotypical people, and it is very important to know that supporting autistic people involves understanding what an experience or situation is like for them and acting accordingly to support and include them. It is about making the world we live in more inclusive for autistic people.

> **EXPERT VOICE: Zahra**
>
> As Omar's mother, I've walked a long, often painful, road. There were countless times where I felt misunderstood by those who didn't know how to approach autism. Autism is not just a diagnosis, but a daily reality.

People with both a learning disability and autism

Learning disability is common in autistic people. About 25% of autistic people have a learning disability, and a further 25% have a borderline learning disability (IQ of 70–85).[11] People who work in services for people with a learning disability and/or autistic people should understand both conditions, as they are likely to be working with at least one individual with a learning disability who is also autistic.

> **EXPERT VOICE: Sam**
>
> It felt great [having my learning disability and autism diagnosis] because it's me. It's important, the need to know what's wrong with me. It's me personally.

The value of inclusion

The vast majority of people with a learning disability and autistic people live in their own homes. They either live on their own, with their families or in supported living homes. Supported living homes are either individual or group homes, where each person has their own tenancy or shared tenancy and paid support from support workers. Some people with a learning disability and/or autistic people live in residential care or nursing care homes, according to their support needs.

All people with a learning disability and autistic people have the right to live lives that are as inclusive as possible in their local communities and society, just as everyone else does, including access to activities, education, employment and health. The value of 'inclusion' is central to supporting people with a learning disability and autistic people in all aspects of their lives[4] and to ensure their overall health and wellbeing.[12]

GLOSSARY

Inclusion – providing equal access to opportunities and resources for people with a learning disability and autistic people, to ensure they are not being marginalised, disadvantaged or excluded.[13]

The value of inclusion will be utilised throughout this book, to demonstrate how all of us, as equal citizens, can include and support people with a learning disability and autistic people more in all aspects of daily life.

It's like looking through a two-way glass. I'm stuck behind on one side looking out. I want to be part of it, but the world's not seeing me and letting me be part of the world. I think that's important because that's how I see my life.

REFLECTION: From integration to inclusion

Alex went to a school for students with a learning disability until he turned eighteen. He now attends a computing course at his local college, with support from his support worker, with whom he sits exclusively during his classes and comfort breaks. With his college placement, Alex has been **integrated** into mainstream further education, but he is still experiencing segregation (exclusion) to some degree.

It is not until Alex spends his class time and breaks with his peers, who are other students on the computing course, and develops friendships with a few of them outside of college hours, that we can say he is being **included.**

This example illustrates the difference between integration and inclusion. It also helps us to think about what we – as equal citizens in society – can do, to include others, and help friendships and support develop naturally.

2 Supporting choices and decision making

A person with a learning disability or an autistic person may require support to make decisions. From day-to-day decisions about what to eat for dinner or what movie to see at the cinema, to more complex decisions about whether or not to sign a tenancy agreement for housing or have surgery for a health issue. It is essential that an individual with a learning disability or an autistic individual is supported to make decisions in such a way that decisions made by or about them reflect their own personal choices.[1]

Having choices is important for making decisions. The more choices a person has, the more opportunities they have to enrich their life and be empowered to make decisions. Can a person with a learning disability or an autistic person make a wrong decision? Well, we all make these at times. Can a person make a decision that involves risk? Yes. Positive, reasonable and informed risks – and countering these risks – also enrich a person's life. For example, Yasmin is looking at pictures in holiday brochures with her support workers. She wants to go on a beach holiday, but her support workers are concerned about taking her wheelchair on to a beach ('What if the wheels get stuck in the sand and the chair topples over, or what if the tide comes in?'). The support workers want to support Yasmin's choice, however, so they find a company online who hire out beach-friendly wheelchairs. Yasmin also decides she wants to try cycling on holiday. The same company has instructors who will take Yasmin out on one of their bikes that has been adapted for wheelchair users.

Decision making and the law

> **GLOSSARY**
>
> **Legal capacity** – the formal ability to hold and exercise rights and duties. Everyone has this right.[2]
>
> **Mental capacity** – the decision-making skills and competencies of a person, which vary from person to person.[2]

There are laws in place throughout the UK that have been enacted to safeguard, without restricting, the rights of people with a learning disability and autistic people to have control over their own lives.[3,4,5] The principles underpinning these Acts can be summarised as follows (allowing for some variation across Northern Ireland, England & Wales and Scotland):

- Individuals are presumed to have capacity unless it can be demonstrated that they lack capacity.

- Individuals must be supported to make decisions, and must have opportunities and encouragement to develop and exercise their capabilities and skills.
- Decisions made with the person must be in their best interests.
- Decisions made with the person must be the least restrictive option for them.
- The individual's wishes, feelings and values must be considered at all times.
- A person has the right to make an unwise decision; this alone does not mean that the person lacks capacity.
- Relevant others (family, friends or carers) should be consulted in the decision-making process, to ensure that a range of perspectives from those who have an interest in the person's wellbeing are considered.

According to these Acts, if a person lacks mental capacity to make an important decision on their own, such as signing a supported housing contract or agreeing to medical treatment, then the person's nearest relative, welfare guardian or attorney, or appointed person (an appointed person is applicable to Northern Ireland only) may decide with them in their best interests as part of the process of their involvement with the supported housing or medical team providing their support or action.[3,4,5] Written proof of an individual's appointed named person will be documented in their care or support plan. Legal decisions, made with individuals in their best interests, must support the person to be involved in the decision as much as they are able to, and must be the least restrictive decision for them. It is fundamental to the rights of a person with a learning disability or an autistic person that 'best interests' means prioritising the wishes and feelings of the person who is at the centre of the decision being made.[2] It is also important to note that capacity is decision specific. For example, the person may be able to make everyday decisions, such as what to wear or eat for dinner, on their own.

EXPERT VOICE: Lizzie

My appointee looks after my money for me. I have to ask my manager or senior support to email my appointee, and he'll say yes or no. I am really pleased that I have got an appointee because if I don't have an appointee, I waste my money. On my debit card, on Tuesday I get paid £40, and on Friday I get paid £50. I have asked for that to happen, so if I blow my money on Tuesday, I get paid on the Friday instead of waiting for the next week. I made that decision.

Advocacy

An advocate is someone who can assist a person with a learning disability or an autistic person to express their views and wishes, and to exercise and uphold their rights. An advocate is often someone who is independent from the person's formal care and support arrangements – a neutral person – but they may also be someone who knows the person well, such as their parent. If you know someone with a learning disability or an autistic person who would benefit from advocacy, then you will be able to find advocacy groups and services for people with a learning disability and/or autistic people in their local area via an online search. Some of these groups or services will also provide advice, assistance and resources to promote self-advocacy to support the person to become more able to speak up for themselves.

Supported decision making

'Supported decision making' is best practice when working with people with a learning disability and autistic people who require support to make decisions. Supported decision making is a process that supports the individual either to decide by themselves or to ensure their will and preferences are at the heart of substitute decision making within the law (for example, guardianship or compulsory treatment orders).[1]

Supported decision making involves the person's friends, family and others within their circle of support, if they wish, to help them participate in and make decisions; at the same time, it ensures that their supporters are not placing any undue influence on their decision making. A person's advocate, if they have one, would also be part of this. Experts, such as a speech and language therapist or a doctor, can also be part of this.

The process involves ensuring that the person has enough time and information to consider options before reaching a decision, and that discussions are held at times and places that are convenient for them. Supported decision making is about utilising communication aids (such as accessible information in easy language and/or pictures and symbols formats) appropriate to the person's needs, when necessary, to aid the person's understanding of their options and the possible outcomes of their decision.[1]

EXPERT VOICE: Zahra

I constantly questioned if I was doing what was best for him. Omar is deeply in his own world, so he hasn't reached the stage of making significant choices for himself. His decisions are limited to daily things, like picking out his clothes or choosing a snack. I want professionals to understand that this is not just about helping children like Omar, but also about supporting parents who bear the immense weight of making critical decisions every single day.

Acquiescence

'Acquiescence' (yes-saying) means to reluctantly accept or agree to something without protest. The term is commonly associated with people with a learning disability and has been used loosely to describe a number of response issues, which can become apparent when asking individuals to answer questions or make choices.[6,7] In truth, communication is a two-way process, and it is necessary for the person asking the questions, or presenting choices, to tailor them to the comprehension abilities and preferred communication style of an individual with a learning disability and to check the person's understanding at various points to ensure that they are expressing their own views or choices.[6] Some of these response issues, and suggestions to overcome them, are presented in Table 2.1.

Table 2.1: Acquiescence and other issues and how to overcome them

Issue	Suggestions
Reluctant acceptance or agreement	Promote choice-making and remind the person frequently that it is their choice. Ensure the person feels included and that what they say or choose is important.

(Continued)

Table 2.1: (Continued)

Issue	Suggestions
Person may not understand	Avoid jargon. Present the questions or information according to the person's preferred communication style (for example, using easy language, pictures or symbols). Break questions or information into smaller chunks and check the person's understanding before moving on. Check the person's understanding by asking them to tell you (or show you) what the words and phrases mean to them.
Tendency to answer 'yes' to all yes/no questions	Ask open-ended questions. If the person finds open-ended questions too difficult to answer, then promote easier choice making instead. For example, 'Here are four pens. What pen colour would you like?'
Suggestibility	Avoid asking leading questions, such as 'You want to go to the park, don't you?'

Issue	Suggestions
Wanting to please the person asking the questions or being submissive.	Ensure the person is comfortable and at ease in the setting. Pay attention to any 'authority figure' dynamics between you and the person. For example, instead of saying 'I am Nurse Jackson' say, 'My name is Karen. I am a nurse'. Be positive and supportive throughout.
Wanting to give the 'correct' answer	Avoid leading questions. Ensure that the person understands that there is no right or wrong answer, but whatever they say or choose is important.

REFLECTION: Tea or coffee?

Example 1a:
Mary: 'Thanks for helping me bring my groceries in from the car, Jamie. I am about to put the kettle on. Do you want a cup of tea?'
Jamie: 'Yes.'
Mary: 'Or do you want a cup of coffee?'
Jamie: 'Yes.'

Example 2a:
George: 'Lee, I am going to make us a cuppa each to drink with the sandwiches we have prepared. Do you want a cup of tea or coffee?'

Lee: 'Coffee.'
George: 'Sorry, I didn't hear you. Did you say you want a cup of coffee or tea?'
Lee: 'Tea.'

In these examples, Jamie and Lee, both of whom have a learning disability, do not seem able to follow what they are being asked; Jamie is saying 'yes' to both questions, and each time, Lee is repeating the last word George said. Mary and George need to adapt their communication, to use fewer words and to ask open-ended questions instead. They may also use visual prompts to aid understanding, such as pointing to a cup, kettle or jar of coffee. Perhaps Jamie and Lee would prefer something other than tea or coffee to drink.

Example 1b:
Mary: 'Thank you for helping. What do you want to drink?'
Jamie: 'Milk.'

Example 2b:
George: 'We have sandwiches to eat. What do you want to drink?'
Lee: 'Tea.'

Autistic people and decision making

Many autistic people have excellent decision-making skills, in terms of their ability to apply reason and make logical decisions.[8] Think for a moment about any autistic characters you are familiar with, portrayed in television programmes or movies, as being able to sort through large volumes of complex information to arrive at an answer or decision. This stereotype of autistic people being 'geniuses', however, is in no way representative of the heterogeneity of autistic people, nor the issues they face and which having to make a decision may pose for them.

Many autistic people – including logical decision makers – experience difficulty making quick decisions on the spot.[9] For example, Philip finds it too difficult to decide what to buy for dinner in a supermarket, particularly as he finds a supermarket a challenging environment to be in. Instead, Philip plans his shopping list before he goes to the supermarket. He also makes sure that he has a plan B for each item he is intending to buy, in case it is out of stock when he gets there (he wants to avoid at all costs an unexpected decision on what to buy as an alternative or coming home empty-handed because he was unable to decide).

Autistic people report several issues that they experience when faced with decision making. These issues include avoiding making decisions (for example, because this will involve a change of routine or having to talk to someone they are not familiar with), finding the decision-making process exhausting or overwhelming (for example, feeling overloaded with information), their sensory needs getting in the way (for example, sensitivity to the environment) and feeling anxious.[9] It is important to be mindful of these potential issues when supporting an autistic person to decide on something; take the following steps to help:

- Ensure the person has as much time as they need to decide.
- Avoid including irrelevant information and reduce the number of choices (for example, provide a choice of two movies to watch, based on the person's known preferences, rather than a choice of eight).
- Provide encouragement and reassurance.
- Address general issues around anxiety.[9]

3

Support in daily life

Supporting people with a learning disability and autistic people in their daily lives requires a commitment to the principles of inclusion and self-determination. Self-determination means having personal autonomy to make decisions – to live a life of choice. These principles underpin the way in which we must provide the right support at the right time to enable people to live a life of their choosing. Based on these principles, in the UK and many other countries, the vast majority of people with a learning disability and autistic people live in their communities – just as everyone else – with varying levels and forms of support from others; this enables them to live in their own homes, to maintain meaningful relationships with friends and family and to be able to engage in activities, including employment.

Individuals with a learning disability and autistic individuals have unique and diverse daily support needs, ranging from getting up to start their day, washing and dressing to preparing a meal or going to a doctor's appointment or on holiday. Individuals are supported across all aspects of these needs in such a way that their individual choices and preferences, wellbeing and independence are promoted.

Personal routines

Personal routines are an important part of daily life. Individuals have wide-ranging supports based on their individual needs and preferences. For example, Zola has a profound learning disability and uses a wheelchair. There is a hoist and shower seat in her home, so her parents can support her to transfer from her bed to her wheelchair to the shower seat or toilet. Ali on the other hand, who has a mild learning disability and is autistic, lives on his own, but he employs a personal assistant to support his travel on a bus to work each morning and afternoon during week days; because the bus is busy it can increase his anxiety making it difficult for him to travel alone.

REFLECTION: Morning routine

Take a few moments to think about your own personal morning routine and preferences. What time do you wake up? Do you have a favourite brand of toothpaste or shower gel that you use? Do you shower before or after breakfast? Do you prefer to use a rough or soft towel to dry yourself? Do you warm your socks on a radiator before putting them on? What do you like to eat for breakfast? Do you listen to the radio in the kitchen or car? Would it affect your mood if you didn't have your favourite toothpaste or ran out of your favourite cereal?

Now, compare your morning routine with that of your friend, colleague or family member (who doesn't live with you). Do they go out for a jog before breakfast? Do they get up earlier or later than you, or hit the snooze button on their alarm clock a few times before getting out of bed? Do they skip breakfast and drink three cups of coffee instead? How would you both feel if you had to swap your morning routines with each other for a week?

This exercise helps you appreciate the importance of respecting an individual's personal needs, preferences and choices throughout the day, right down to the minute details of their favourite items, time needed, textures, scents, tastes, and sounds.

Autistic people and routines

For some autistic people, routines, and the sequences of those routines, are especially important. The familiarity of their routines helps them to cope with a world that can seem to them to be unpredictable and confusing.[1] We exist in a world that is focused on the needs of neurotypical people, which can exclude or fail to recognise the needs of some members of our society. Some autistic people cope in this neurotypical world by having routines that make sense to them, perhaps accommodating their sensory needs or their need for predictability. Yet sometimes change is unavoidable (for example, bereavement) or potentially beneficial (for example, going on holiday). Strategies to support an autistic person to adapt to change include the following:

- Planning for change, providing the person with as much information as possible beforehand to help them prepare.
- Where a change is predicted, asking the person what they need to adapt to this change.
- Involving others in the change.
- Sequencing and the use of visual aids to show the person what is happening, in what order and when.

It is important to be aware that autistic individuals can experience anxiety around changes to their routines. Be mindful to avoid such anxiety, by keeping the person involved and at the centre of any decisions about change; also check for signs of anxiety, offer reassurance, and assist the person by providing them with the chance to ask questions about change, as well as giving them the time and support to express how they are feeling.[1]

Person-centred thinking and support

Being 'person-centred' means putting the person at the centre of the support provided. It ensures that the person's needs, wishes and preferences drive what their support should be. It is broader than just what we do in terms of providing support; it is a way of thinking.

Person-centred thinking is a set of values that ensure the person is respected, included and valued.[2] The core principles of person-centred support include:

- Good communication systems with the person and across the services that support them.
- Viewing the person's family and loved ones as partners in their care and support.
- Being compassionate and seeing things from the person's point of view.
- Support is dignified and sensitive to people's personal needs and preferences.[2]

EXPERT VOICE: Kriss

[Stephen] got to know when I was having my good days and when I was having my bad days. He used to meet me in the middle. If he came in and said, 'Right Kriss, we've got this to do today', and I was like, 'Do we have to?', he'd say, 'Well, let's do one bit and then we'll have a break or we'll do something else'. He used to say, 'Well, if you do your washing up and put everything away, then we'll stop and have a cup of tea, listen to a musical, have a chat or go out for a coffee'.

Person-centred active support (PCAS)

An emphasis on person-centred active support (PCAS) for people with a learning disability and autistic people is paramount, as it enables them to participate, irrespective of their level of disability. PCAS is focused on achieving the right level of support for the individual to ensure the have opportunities for meaningful engagement and inclusion, leading to a better quality of life because of a better quality of support. While observing the support provided at one of the first community-based group homes for people with a learning disability in England during the 1980s, it was recognised that people with a learning disability were often excluded from having any meaningful involvement in their own lives.[3,4] For example, everyday activities, such as cooking meals and shopping for food, were done for individuals rather than with them. This was later referred to as a 'hotel model' of support, where the support provided was, in fact, *dis*empowering people to have any control over their lives.[5] PCAS empowers people to be active and involved.

GLOSSARY

Meaningful engagement – to be considered meaningful, an engagement should align with the person's values, promote a sense of accomplishment and generate positive emotions. It should also foster connections with others and create a sense of community, while promoting a sense of autonomy.[6]

PCAS has four key components:[7]

1. **Every moment has potential** is about seeing and identifying real and naturally occurring

opportunities for people to be meaningfully involved. For instance, it looks at the things we all need to do as part of our home life, or at the activities that we enjoy or seek to do, at home and in the community, including interactions with all the people around us, and encourages consideration of how the person might be included in these moments right now. Examples include being on first-name terms and exchanging pleasantries with a local shopkeeper, doing the food shopping, answering the door when someone visits and knowing the neighbours.

2. **Graded assistance to ensure success** is about providing the right level and type of support at the right time: too much and they will be over-supported, which means they don't have the opportunity to learn and develop; too little and they will be unsuccessful, meaning the person may be reluctant to be involved next time. For example, Daisy is being actively supported to cook pasta for dinner. She starts by learning where to find the dried pasta in the food cupboard and pouring a cup full into a pan of water. Over time, she will become involved in preparing all aspects of a pasta meal.

3. **Maximising choice and control** values the person's views on what to do, when and with whom, rather than having a focus on doing things according to someone else's wishes, a timetable or a daily planner. The ways in which many

supported people with a learning disability and autistic people spend their time can be dictated by the people providing the support (for example, in supported living or residential care settings). PCAS puts the person at the centre of decisions made about what they do and when.

4. **Little and often** is recognising that everything that happens throughout the day is made up of smaller parts or steps. Seeing things this way enables us to identify how people can get involved in activities in a way that works for them. Some examples of this include the person dipping in and out of an activity rather than be expected to complete the whole thing, being supported in a way that builds on what the person can do, and working at a pace that keeps the person interested and involved.

Families as experts

In the UK, the majority of people with a learning disability and autistic people live at home with their families. Family members should be treated as experts on the support needs of their relative. They have extensive knowledge and understanding of their relative's history, preferences, values and needs. It is important to work in partnership with families as experts in designing and evaluating support. In addition, family members and supporters can be strong advocates for a person, especially when the individual is unable to express their preferences or needs, to ensure that the person's rights and wishes are respected.[8]

> **EXPERT VOICE: Zahra**
>
> Every day with Omar is unpredictable. What seems simple for other children can be a mountain for him. My heart aches for the days when I couldn't find the right help. Families need professionals who understand how essential proper support is for the everyday battles we face.

Supporting young people

People's daily support needs, and their support services, change at different stages of their lives. For most people who use support services, the provision of services change during their lifetime from child and young person to adult services. This includes, for example, the transition from school to college or employment, and the transition from paediatric to adult healthcare. Transitions can be particularly stressful, fragmented and isolating for the person and their family, and as such the following principles are important in planning their ongoing support:

- Listen to the wishes and feelings of the young person, and put them at the centre of planning and decision making.

- Recognise that young people and their families are experts on their own needs and the services they require.
- Use person-centred planning to assess the young person's needs, and facilitate access to both specialist and mainstream community supports, according to their needs.
- Create and encourage opportunities for the person to live an ordinary life as a citizen in their local community.[8]

> **EXPERT VOICE: Vicky**
>
> I am a happy person. I like having everyone around me as friends. My support staff are kind and helpful to talk to. My support staff help me with cooking and everything, just support me in the kitchen. [In the past when I was around grumpy staff], I would just tell them to leave me alone and go into my bedroom.

Supporting older adults

For people with a learning disability and autistic people who require support, their support needs continue to change throughout their lives. We are an ageing UK population and planning for the future is especially important for adults with a learning disability and autistic adults.

Many adults live with their families, who themselves are getting older and who may not always be able to provide care and support. For example, around 40% of adults with a learning disability who live at home with their families live with a parent aged 60 years old or over (33% live with a parent aged 70 years or over).[9] Advanced care and support planning is essential, as it supports the individual to anticipate grief and bereavement, as well as future and end-of-life care and support.[10]

Assistive technology

Assistive technology refers to any equipment, product or service that a person with a learning disability or an autistic person may use to aid and empower their everyday life. Examples are:

- Posture and mobility – an electric wheelchair, a hoist or a stair lift.
- Daily living aids – a cooker guard, raised toilet seat, a visual timer or hand rails.
- Digital – communication, mind-mapping or health-maintaining software.

Autistic people may also use aids to support their sensory needs and/or to reduce anxiety, such as sound block headphones, specific clothing and stress balls or fidget toys.

If you are supporting someone who would benefit from assistive technology, request an assessment from their local health and social care service, who will signpost them to the most appropriate service to provide this support (for example, physiotherapy, occupational therapy or speech and language therapy).

It is important to ensure that any prescribed aids and adaptations are being used correctly, with regular maintenance checks and training on their use. Non-use or misuse of some aids and adaptations can lead to accidents or injury.[11] The correct use of aids and adaptations can also significantly enhance people's life experiences.

Inclusive communication with people with a learning disability

Communication between people is an essential part of everyday life, enabling individuals to give and receive information, to express opinions, emotions, needs and choices, and to be included. Communication is more than spoken and written words; it also involves non-verbal communication (for example, facial expressions and body language), expressed emotions (for example, crying), gestures (such as pointing or nodding), the senses (for example, hearing a train before it arrives at a train station) and other non-written forms of communication (such as pictures, charts and symbols). Even the way in which we speak communicates more than the words alone can express. For example, if a person is animated, speaking quickly and loudly, they may be expressing excitement. As we go through life and interact with each other, we learn to communicate according to social and cultural norms. For example, whispering in a library or shaking our heads to communicate that we mean no or don't agree; in contrast, in India, for instance, head wobbling or shaking can mean the opposite, in that the person is communicating yes or that they do agree.

People with a learning disability often have communication needs, which vary from individual to individual. For example, whereas some people are able to speak, write and count (for example, when handling money), other people cannot read, formulate sounds rather than words and communicate more using facial expressions and gestures. When you are interacting and communicating with an individual, it is important to be aware of and responsive to their individual communication needs and adapt your communication with them accordingly. It is also crucial that society as a whole champions inclusive communication for people with a learning disability, which means providing and sharing information in such a way that everyone can understand.

Expressive and receptive communication

Spoken communication as an interaction between two people is both expressive and receptive. One person is expressing an opinion, instruction or piece of information, and the other person is being receptive in understanding the other person's point of view, the instruction or the information they are being given. Individuals with a learning disability may have communication needs around expressive and receptive communication. For example, a person may find it difficult to formulate words to express how they are feeling or what they need at that particular moment, so they may rely more on expressions or gestures to communicate this. Alternatively, a person may find it difficult to follow what another person is saying to them and asking them to do, so the other person should speak more slowly to them, using fewer and easier words to facilitate understanding.

People with a learning disability have a condition that affects their general intelligence,[1] so it is important to pay close attention to adapting your communication with each person to facilitate their understanding and to check that they have understood. Some people with a learning disability may not communicate verbally or may use few words, but this does not mean that they do not understand what you are saying when you are speaking with them. Conversely, some people with a learning disability may be very expressive in their verbal communication, but they may be expressing more than they understand. Receptive language and expressive language are not dependent on each other.

Communication needs

EXPERT VOICE: Sam

Just because I have a learning disability, don't speak to me like I am five years old. Not only does it make me feel awkward, it makes it more difficult for me to talk back – it's not how I am.

People with a learning disability prefer others to communicate with them on a one-to-one basis, face-to-face, so they can concentrate on what is being said, as well as facial expressions, body language and gestures. They also find it is better for someone to talk with them slowly and clearly, using words that are easily understood.[2] In terms of facilitating and checking understanding, give a person small amounts of information at a time, and then give them time to process this information. Check the person's understanding with them before moving on to the next thing being discussed. For example, ask them to repeat back to you what you have said in their own words, and ask them if they have any questions before moving on to the next thing.

EXPERT VOICE: Sam

Give me time to think. If someone asks me something and I am struggling, I feel pressure. If they think I need to give them an answer now, it can make it more difficult. Remain silent until I say something, or break it down for me to make it easier to understand.

Here are ten tips for being sensitive and responsive to the communication needs of people with a learning disability.[2]

1. Find a quiet place to communicate without distractions. Ensure the person is comfortable in this setting by paying attention to the environment

(for example, ensuring there is adequate lighting for a person who has a visual impairment).

2. Ask open-ended questions instead of closed yes or no questions to ensure the person has an opportunity to express their needs, wishes and choices. Bearing in mind that people with a learning disability can be more prone to acquiescence and suggestibility, do not ask leading questions (for example, 'You are tired and you want to go home early, don't you?').

3. Check with the person that you understand what they are telling you (for example, 'You are feeling sore, is that right? Can you point and show me where you are feeling sore?').

4. Go with the person if they want to show you something. Sometimes it is easier for them to take you and show you what they mean, rather than trying to explain it verbally.

5. Give the person your full attention and pay attention to how they are communicating with you, using their facial expressions, body language and gestures.

6. Use gestures and facial expressions (for example, if you are asking the person if they feel happy or sad, smile then frown to reinforce what you are saying).

7. Take your time and don't rush. People with a learning disability often require time and patience to process information, as well as time to think about what they want to say and time to communicate with you. Interrupting the person, talking for them or finishing their words for them

are not at all helpful and are likely to cause frustration and stress or leave the person feeling ignored or excluded.

8. Be aware that some people find it easier to understand information, make choices and express themselves by using pictures or symbols. Drawing may also be helpful for the person, even if you do not see yourself as being artistic.

9. Be aware that some people find it easier to communicate using real objects (objects of reference), although photos and pictures can still help too.

10. Remember that people with a learning disability often have a supporter (relative or support worker) who knows them well and can help facilitate communication with them. However, when the person's supporter is present, be sure to always direct your questions to the person with a learning disability, so that you include them at all times.

GLOSSARY

Information-carrying word – the word that gives specific meaning or instruction in a sentence. For example, if you show someone a plate of biscuits and say, 'Would you like a biscuit?', the information-carrying word is 'biscuit'. As the word, as well as your tone and gesture, coupled with the visual plate of biscuits, gives a reasonable representation of what you are asking/offering the person, many of the other words are redundant.[3] Bear this in mind when you are communicating with people with a learning disability. Use relevant information-carrying words, fewer redundant words, and to avoid confusion do not use too many information-carrying words in the same sentence.

Augmentative and alternative communication (AAC)

Augmentative and alternative communication (AAC) is a 'total communication' approach, which is directed towards ensuring positive and inclusive communication with individuals who do not use speech or would benefit from other strategies to support their verbal communication. A total communication approach involves using and accepting all types of communication equally, not just speech. This includes facial expressions, body language, gestures, signs, sounds, symbols, written words, pictures, photos, objects of reference and assistive technology.[4]

GLOSSARY

Object of reference – an object that has a particular meaning, which can be used as a communication aid to refer to a person, object, location or event. For example, a football is associated with playing football and inflatable arm bands can represent going to the swimming pool.[5]

AAC includes Makaton, which is based on British Sign Language (BSL). Four important examples of Makaton signs are toilet (Figure 4.1), home (two hands in the shape of a roof), hungry (rubbing the stomach) and pain (holding a shaking hand where it hurts).[6] Many people with a learning disability use Makaton to assist communication, and the signs are often easy to pick up. For example, when a person with a learning disability goes into a café and makes a C sign with their fingers, followed by a gesture to demonstrate drinking, it doesn't take the barista long to understand that the person would like a cup of coffee.[6] It is worthwhile visiting the Makaton charity website (see Resources) to learn more about Makaton and access free resources. Why don't you learn how to sign your name to a person on their or your hand using Makaton alphabet signs?

Visual aids and supports, such as pictorial timetables, are often used with people with a learning disability, usually with easy words included. Visual supports help with the person's attention, learning, retention of information, communication and expression. Visual supports can help to:

- Provide structure and routine while supporting understanding.
- Manage transitions and move from one activity to another.
- Reduce worry and anxiety, as the person is helped to understand what is happening next.

- Build confidence and encourage independence.
- Provide opportunities to interact with others.

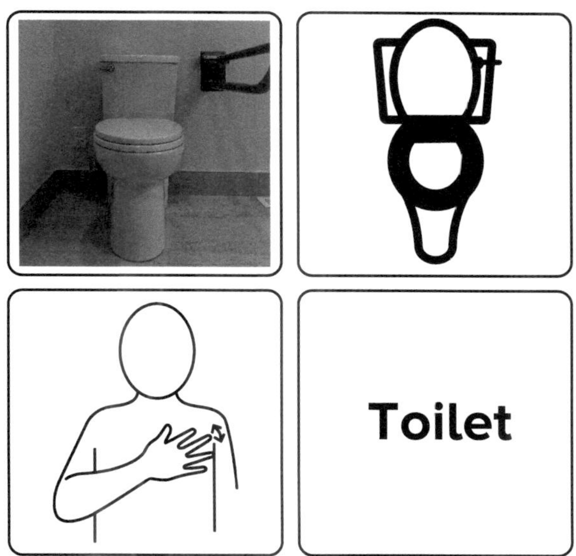

Figure 4.1: Toilet picture, symbol, Makaton sign and word. *Source:* Makaton Symbols and Signs © 2025 The Makaton Charity, makaton.org

Figure 4.2 is an example of a visual timetable using symbols and easy words. When each activity has finished, the person can even take the symbol off their timetable, and place it in a 'finished' box.

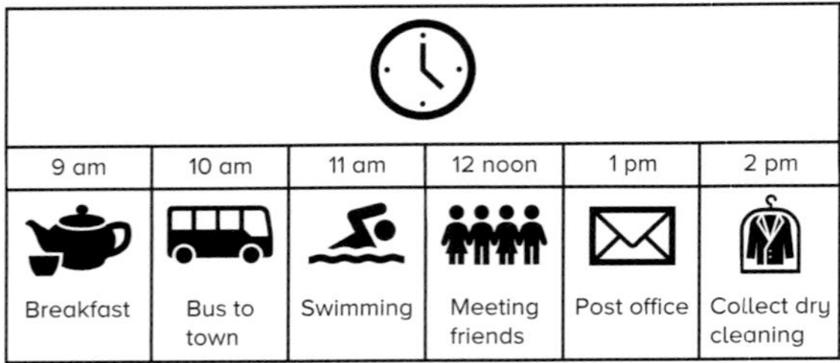

Figure 4.2: Visual timetable.

Another useful example is a visual pain scale (Figure 4.3), which can be used with a person to determine whether or not they are experiencing pain and, if so, to what extent. It is important, however, to use this visual aid alongside awareness of potential symptoms and other ways the person may communicate pain (for example, facial expressions) to avoid misinterpretation. Emoji scales are even better when they are in colour and incorporate a traffic light system, where 1 is green and 6 is red.

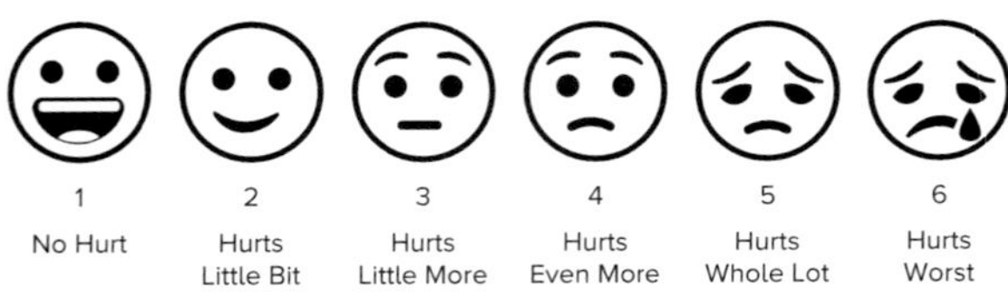

Figure 4.3: Visual pain scale.

Tangible objects of reference are extremely useful for assisting communication with people with a learning disability, as these are items the person can touch, hold and utilise. Objects of reference are used to:

* Assist memory (representing activities or events the person has participated in or done before)
* Aid understanding (by giving the person relevant objects to associate with understanding)
* Enable anticipation of events (by planning ahead and associating objects with what the person is going to participate in)
* Aid expression (by enabling the person to use familiar objects to make choices or requests).

EXPERT VOICE: Marion

We held a swimming costume which had chlorine on it so that Laura could smell it, and know that she was going to the swimming pool.

Accessible information

All health and social care services in the UK are required to provide accessible information for people who use them.[7] Accessible information refers to providing information in accessible formats, using easy language, pictures and symbols. A guide to making information accessible is listed for you in the Resources section (p. 119).

REFLECTION: Accessible information practice

Think about an activity that is upcoming for you this week or month. It could be something as mundane as visiting the dentist or returning a parcel at a Post Office, or something you are looking forward to, such as meeting a friend for lunch or going to a music concert. Write down all of the steps to this activity (for example, travelling to the dentist, sitting in the waiting room, being seen by the dentist and waiting a couple of hours before eating after a filling). Once you have done that, practise using easy words, symbols and pictures to produce the same information in an accessible format. What about objects of reference? Are there any tangible objects you could use to communicate this activity/event to a person with communication needs?

5 Inclusive communication with autistic people

As inclusive communication involves providing and sharing information in such a way that everyone understands, including neurodivergent people, it is important to develop a working knowledge and understanding of how to adapt and enhance your communication when supporting and interacting with autistic people. In order to be able to do this, you must first be aware of and sensitive to how autistic people process information and communicate.

Processing information and communication

Autistic people tend to process information and communicate in the following ways:[1,2]

- **Sarcasm and figurative language:** Autistic people often do not use figurative language, such as metaphors and euphemisms, in their everyday communication. For example, when another person says, 'It's raining cats and dogs', an autistic person may interpret the language literally and think, 'I am confused. Is it really raining cats and dogs?' Autistic people may also not recognise subtleties in social communication, such as sarcasm, innuendo and humour.

- **Sensory information:** Autistic people process sensory information differently. As most environments are designed around the needs of neurotypical people, autistic people can find it difficult to process sensory information, particularly in loud or cluttered environments, and may experience sensory overload. This can include, for example, finding touch or sensations on their skin painful, being unable to filter or drown out background noises, finding noises they hear painful and overwhelming, and being unable to process heavily patterned textiles (such as carpets or wallpaper) and bright lights. In contrast, some individuals with autism are hyposensitive to processing sensory information, preferring loud noises, bright lights and colours, and not recognising sensations such as hunger or pain.
- **Social cues:** Autistic people may be less likely to pick up on the social cues of others, such as facial expressions and body language, although many autistic people use their own facial expressions and body language effectively to communicate.
- **Speech patterns:** Autistic people may be less likely to follow conventional speech patterns, for example, using shorter sentences (to get to a point more directly). Some autistic people

may be repetitive in their speech, repeating the same words and phrases (known as echolalia), or they may use memorised speech (known as scripting).

- **Interpretation of norms:** Autistic people can interpret norms and customs (for example, shaking hands when greeting someone) in social communication differently or can find them difficult or uncomfortable. For example, an autistic person may find eye contact uncomfortable or distracting, and prefer to avoid it or make only fleeting glances when they are talking with someone.

GLOSSARY

Alexithymia ('having no words for emotion') – 50% of autistic people find it difficult to identify and interpret their emotions or how they are feeling internally.[3] This does not mean at all that autistic people do not experience emotions or that all autistic people are alike. Indeed, many autistic people have strong emotional intelligence in terms of managing their emotions and being empathetic towards others.

It is important to be sensitive and empathetic to the differences in how autistic people may interpret and process information, and to ensure you and others are not making negative and mistaken assumptions.[4]

For example, the person is not being intentionally aloof or rude because they are not communicating with you and others in a way that people living in a world that is geared more towards neurotypical people are accustomed to. We all need to be aware of our own bias and assumptions about people's intentions so that they do not become a barrier to communication. Embracing difference and diversity is conductive to living in an inclusive society.

Communication strengths

Autistic people have unique ways of experiencing the world, meaning that many autistic individuals have particular communication strengths:[2]

- **Directness and honesty:** Due to literal communication, many autistic individuals communicate directly and honestly. Such attributes are highly valued for personal integrity.
- **Attention to details:** An intense focus on particular interests or details means that an autistic person can be especially technically-minded or analytical and can pick up on finer details and points that others may miss.
- **Focus and perseverance:** An autistic person's ability to focus on topics of interest is in itself a strength.
- **Unique perspectives:** An autistic person's ability to see things differently, or 'think outside of

the box', can offer new insights and different solutions when problem-solving.

- **Logical approach:** Many autistic individuals have strong reasoning skills and can present arguments in a clear and logical manner.
- **Creativity and innovation:** Autism is related to having a strong imagination and unique thinking patterns.
- **Technical and visual communication:** Many autistic individuals excel in technical and visual communication and have a particular aptitude for skills such as computer programming, graphic design and data visualisation (such as graphs and charts).

STEP IT UP communication guide

Autistic people are individuals and vary greatly according to their individual support and communication needs. For example, whereas one autistic person can be highly intelligent and have a masterful grasp of spoken and written language, another autistic person can have no verbal communication at all and must rely on other forms of communication, such as picture cards, communication boards and gestures. Figure 5.1 is an example of a communication board for an autistic person ('turn' refers to the person knowing when it is their turn when interacting with other people).

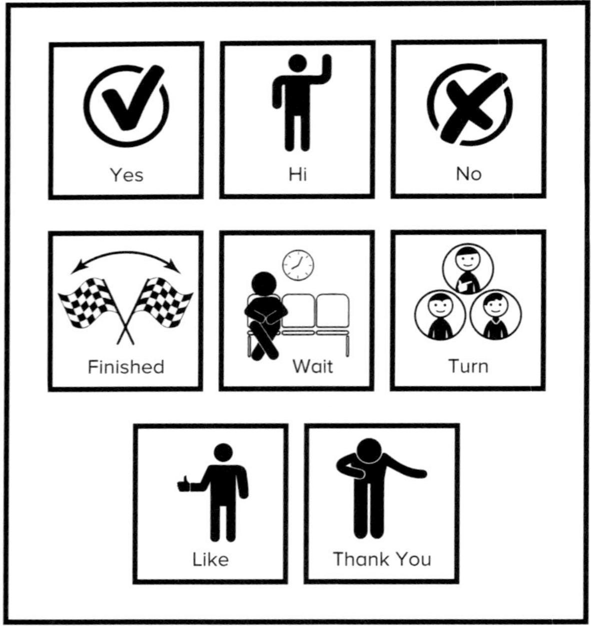

Figure 5.1: Communication board example.

The STEP IT UP communication guide[5] is a very useful guide for communicating with autistic people with communication support needs (Table 5.1).

Table 5.1: The STEP IT UP communication guide

Simple and direct questions	Ask the person one question at a time. Use easy words and avoid jargon. For example, instead of saying 'Do you feel nauseous? You are pyrexical', say 'You have a fever. Do you feel sick?'
Take your time	Be patient and wait for the person to process the information and answer. Allow as much time as necessary for communication.
Explain to enable understanding	Explain everything to the person to ensure their understanding of what is happening and what will happen next and to ensure they are happy/comfortable/in agreement. Routines, particularly the sequence of these routines, can be very important to an autistic person.
Precise language	Say exactly what you mean and be descriptive. Avoid metaphors and euphemisms. For example, instead of saying 'She has a heart of gold', say 'She is a kind person'.
Include carers	Be aware that the person's supporter (for example, their relative) knows the person well and can guide and facilitate your communication with them.

(Continued)

Table 5.1: *(Continued)*

Touch and feel first	Provide tangible objects of reference that the person can touch, feel and become familiar with. If you are using objects with the person, advise them beforehand of any sensations (for example, 'This needle will prick your skin. I can put cream on your arm first to numb the pain. The cream will feel cold on your skin when I apply it.'). Be truthful (for example, don't say something won't hurt if you know it will).
Understand my differences	Be aware of and understand the potential communication differences between an autistic person and a neurotypical person. For example, an autistic person may find some things painful on their skin (such as some clothing fabrics or shower water), or they may find it challenging to express that they are experiencing pain. Also, do not assume the person's behaviour is normal for them (for example, appearing disruptive or aggressive). Exhaust all possible reasons for their behaviour.

Prepare a low sensory environment	Use a quiet room with minimal distractions. Avoid bright lighting and noisy, cluttered places. Provide noise-reducing headphones (ear defenders) as necessary.

STEP IT UP is an equally useful guide for communicating with people with a learning disability, as well as other neurodivergent groups of people.

Communication tips

As well as the STEP IT UP guide, other tips for communicating positively and effectively with autistic people are as follows:[3,6]

1. Use the person's name when you are speaking with them, so that they know you are talking to them, and as a cue for them to respond.
2. Be aware that the person may be more comfortable communicating with one person at a time, so do not crowd them.
3. Understand and respect that the person may avoid eye contact with you; they are still listening to you and communicating in other ways.
4. Understand and respect that the person may find it difficult to read and respond to your facial expressions and body language. At the same time, remember that augmentative and alternative

communication (AAC) encompasses all forms of communication, and there are many other forms of communication available; facial expressions and body language are only a part of that.

5. If the person is being repetitive in their speech or fidgeting with their hands or a toy, do not interrupt this. This is known as 'stimming' and the person is doing this to calm themselves.

6. If the person reads, they may prefer written rather than spoken information.

Picture exchange communication system (PECS)

Between 25% and 30% of autistic people do not speak at all, or speak a few words only.[7] Picture exchange communication systems (PECS) are often used with autistic people as a communication tool. A PECS uses a series of picture cards, which a person can use to exchange for whatever they want or need at a particular time (for example, exchanging a picture of a duck to go to the park and feed the birds at the duck pond). Over time the person increases the number of cards they use and learns to use a combination of cards together (for example, going to the park with my brother), as well as using cards in the context of sentences (for example, 'I want …'). PECS are very useful for developing the person's communication, as well as their confidence and self-esteem.

EXPERT VOICE: Zahra

The hardest part of raising Omar has been knowing that he's trying to tell me something, but the words don't come. I've had to learn to read his eyes, his gestures, his silences. It's crucial that health and social care professionals learn how to connect with autistic people who communicate beyond words.

REFLECTION: Euphemisms and metaphors

Over the course of the next day or couple of days, observe your social communication interactions and make a mental note, or write down, all of the euphemisms, metaphors, sarcastic comments, for example, that you and the people you are interacting with use in your everyday conversations (include everyone, from your local shopkeeper and postman, to your close friends and family, and your colleagues). Once you have completed your list, review these sentences/phrases/figures of speech, and spend time thinking how you would rephrase them to explain their literal meaning to an autistic person. For example, 'I am thirsty' instead of 'I am dying for a drink'.

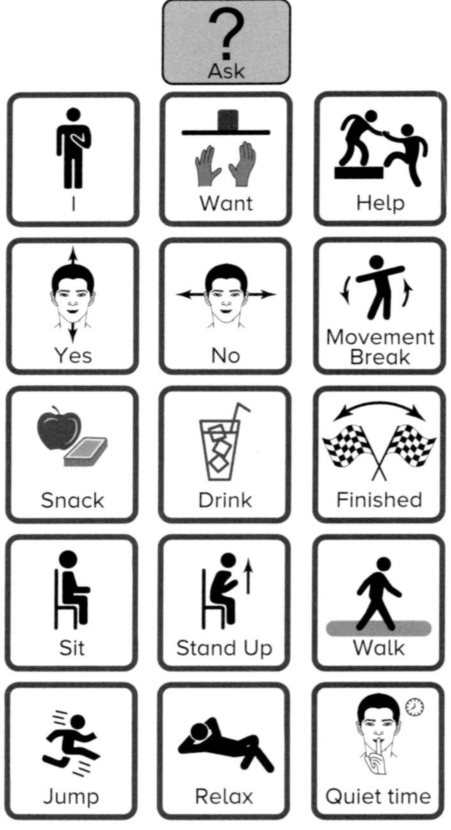

Figure 5.2: A PECS example.

Physical health and wellbeing

People with a learning disability and autistic people have different patterns of health from the general population. These include lower life expectancy, different causes of death and higher rates of physical and mental health conditions. Multi-morbidity, which means having two or more long-term health conditions, is also common.[1] It is important to be aware of the specific health needs of people with a learning disability and autistic people to ensure their needs are being met. It is also important that health and social care addresses health inequalities experienced by people with a learning disability and autistic people.

GLOSSARY

Health inequalities – differences in health (for example, life expectancy) between different groups in society, which are avoidable, unfair and systematic.[2] The reasons for these inequalities are complex but include, for example, discrimination, lack of access to services or lack of accessible information.

A systematic health inequality can be, for example, when government funding is prioritised to prevent and treat health conditions most commonly experienced by the general population (to benefit as many people as possible), but not prioritised to prevent and treat health conditions more commonly experienced by people with a learning disability or autistic people (who represent a smaller percentage of the UK population). Funding allocation should also include tailored prevention and treatment initiatives for minority groups within the population.

Another example can be a woman not being routinely offered cervical screening because she is assumed, by her healthcare provider, to not be sexually active because she has a learning disability. To address this health inequality, the healthcare provider should offer cervical screening to all women without discrimination, provide accessible information about cervical smear tests and make any adjustments that are reasonable and necessary to ensure access to health screening.

Life expectancy and causes of death

People with a learning disability and autistic people tend not to live as long as other people. In 2022, the average age of death for men and women with a learning disability was 63 years, compared to 82 years for men and 86 years for women in the general population. In the same year, the average age of death for autistic men was 77 years and 75 years for autistic women.[3] The three main causes of death for people with a learning disability are cardiovascular conditions (including heart disease), respiratory conditions and cancer;[3] the three main causes of death for the general population are dementia, heart disease and respiratory conditions.[4] In addition, people in the general population are more likely to experience lung, breast, prostate, oral and cervical cancers, whereas people with a learning disability are more likely to experience cancer of the digestive organs or testicular cancer in men.[5]

Autistic people are more likely to die from suicide or accidents, particularly drowning for autistic children.[3,6] Autistic children, especially those experiencing over-stimulation, can wander off (known as elopement) and be drawn to water because of its calming effects. Water safety, including swimming lessons, is an important consideration for autistic children.

Alarmingly, around 42% of deaths of people with learning disability (including those who are also autistic) are avoidable deaths. An avoidable death means that death could have been prevented if the person had received treatment in time that was effective.[3] It is paramount, therefore, when working with someone who has a high level of support needs, to be vigilant and to pay close attention to how the person may communicate pain or discomfort, and to be alert to possible early symptoms of illness.

Constipation is an example of a common health complaint that can be treated with increased fibre in the diet, laxatives or abdominal massage. Untreated constipation, however, can be agonising and can lead to the person's bowel becoming so full of faeces that it may burst and cause death.[7] When you are working with someone with high support needs, keep a bowel chart to monitor their bowel habits (such as frequency and faeces texture) to ensure and maintain bowel health.

Physical health conditions

> **EXPERT VOICE: Sam**
>
> I wasn't feeling very well, sinuses or something. I went to see if they could give me some medication. My mum went with me. The doctor got me involved. She spoke to me individually. She didn't turn to my mum and say, 'Is that alright?'. That made me feel really comfy, chatting and that.

People with a learning disability and autistic people experience a number of physical health conditions more commonly, either in general or within specific conditions. For example, generally speaking, people with a learning disability are more prone to having impacted ear wax, and people with Down syndrome even more so because they have narrower ear canals. Some of the physical health conditions commonly experienced by people with a learning disability and autistic people are listed in Tables 6.1 and 6.2.[8–13] When you are supporting people with a specific learning disability condition, such as Down syndrome, it is worthwhile sourcing trusted and reliable websites for more information about their particular health needs.

Table 6.1: Physical health conditions commonly experienced by people with a learning disability

Physical health condition	Proportion of people with a learning disability affected
Visual impairment	47%
Obesity	Between 35% and 41%
Epilepsy	Between 34% and 52%
Constipation	34%
Urinary incontinence	32%
Ataxic/gait disorders	30%
Hearing impairment	Between 27% and 35%
Bowel incontinence	23%
Nail disorder (for example, in-growing toenail)	23%
Epidermal thickening/ xerosis	21%
Cerebral palsy and other paralytic conditions	Between 19% and 29%
Osteoporosis	Between 18% and 41%

Table 6.2: Physical health conditions commonly experienced by autistic people

Physical health condition	Proportion of autistic people affected
Sleep problems	50%
Epilepsy	33%
Near sightedness (short sight)	31%
Irritable bowel syndrome (IBS)	25%
Astigmatism (eye condition that causes, for example, blurred vision)	25%
Migraine	23%
Eczema	21%
Gastric reflux	20%
Chronic constipation	10%
Chronic diarrhoea	8%

Epilepsy is very common among people with a learning disability and autistic people. Epilepsy management and support plans are important for individuals with epilepsy. These plans include seizure activity monitoring (types and frequency), regular reviews of anti-epileptic medication, and identifying and avoiding factors known to trigger the person's seizures (such as lack of sleep, stress, drinking alcohol or photosensitivity). Sudden unexpected death in epilepsy (SUDEP) occurs when the heart or breathing stops during or after a seizure. SUDEP is rare – occurring in 3–9 in every 1000 people with a learning disability (including those who are also autistic) with epilepsy[14] – but risk factors associated with SUDEP do include poorly controlled seizures and seizures during the night.[15] Taking antiepileptic medication as prescribed and monitoring seizures during the night (for example, using an epilepsy alarm or monitor) counter these risks.

People with a learning disability and autistic people are twice as likely to experience injuries from accidents (such as falls, drowning, burns and scalds, and choking) compared to people in the general population.[13] Risk assessments, promoting opportunities to live full and meaningful but safe lives, are also important.

People with a learning disability and autistic people should not miss routine appointments to maintain their health and wellbeing, and they must be supported to follow treatment and advice between appointments. For example, if the person has prescription glasses or hearing aids, ensure they are wearing the correct ones (not an old pair found at the back of a drawer) and that they are cleaned regularly and are in working order at all times (for example, battery checks for hearing aids).

Health checks

The optimum way to promote and maintain the health and wellbeing of people with a learning disability and autistic people is for each individual to have an annual check-up (known as a health check) via their general practice (GP). If you are supporting individuals with appointments for annual health checks, it is important that they do not miss these appointments. Health checks, for example, can identify and treat health conditions not previously diagnosed. If you are supporting individuals who do not have appointments for annual health checks, speak with each person's healthcare team to request this.

Lifestyle

Obesity is common among people with a learning disability, particularly those who have limited opportunities for regular exercise and/or those with unhealthy diets. Unhealthy lifestyles can lead to further health complications, such as type 2 diabetes. People with a learning disability, however, are diverse, and some individuals with a learning disability are underweight or have special diets (for example, percutaneous endoscopic gastronomy (PEG) tube feeding).

People with a learning disability and autistic people should be supported to make informed choices towards healthy lifestyles. Lifestyle factors that can impact on a person's health and wellbeing refer not only to exercise and diet, but also smoking, alcohol, recreational drugs, sleep, stress, loneliness and screen time on smartphones or tablets.

Polypharmacy

Polypharmacy (being prescribed multiple different drugs at the same time) is common among people with a learning disability and autistic people, who have high rates of co-occurring physical and mental health conditions. Regular medication reviews (for example, to monitor possible side-effects) are important for these individuals. Individuals should also have opportunities to explore non-pharmaceutical treatments for health conditions. For example, prebiotics or cranberry juice can promote a healthy bladder and reduce the risk of developing urinary tract infections (UTIs). Positive behaviour support (PBS) plans can reduce the number and dosage of psychotropic drugs (drugs that affect behaviour, mood, thoughts and perceptions) being prescribed.[16]

Sexual health

People with a learning disability and autistic people have the same human rights as everyone else, including the right to marry and have children. However, adults with a learning disability, and autistic adults with support needs, have not been found to have the same freedoms as everyone else, due to concerns around consent, vulnerability, possible exploitation and, in some instances, infantilising attitudes towards them (treating them as though they are still children).[18]

People with a learning disability and autistic people who choose to should be supported to have romantic and sexual relationships that are not coercive, exploitative or abusive. This support should include having social opportunities to meet prospective partners. It is also important that people with a learning disability and autistic people have the same equal access to sexual health services as everyone else (for example, breast screening and smear tests, testicular cancer awareness, family planning, menopause support and gender diversity support and services).

> **EXPERT VOICE: Brett**
>
> I like [the] emphasis on not over-coddling, such as sex lives as something we should be allowed to pursue.

Diagnostic overshadowing

Diagnostic overshadowing occurs when a person's symptoms or health issues are wrongly assumed to be part of their disability. It is important to be aware of this to ensure that possible symptoms (such as limping, slurred speech, aggression or being slow to respond or react) and health issues are not ignored or missed. Catherine, for example, was experiencing toilet accidents (urinary incontinence) and was hiding wet clothes in her bedroom because she felt embarrassed and ashamed. She had just moved into a new nursing home, and her nursing team assumed that her toileting issues were due to her learning disability. This was not the case at all, as previously she was fully continent. Catherine's community learning disability nurse ruled out any physical causes (for example, urinary tract infection) and then supported the nursing team to develop a personal toileting plan with her, which included wearing a toilet alarm watch to remind her to void in a toilet at regular intervals throughout the day. A few months later Catherine was no longer experiencing toilet accidents.

David has Down syndrome. He tripped going down an escalator in a department store and the store staff called an emergency first responder for him. The first responder who attended to David wasn't sure if his slow speech was how he normally spoke or whether it was a symptom of concussion. He did not have any obvious sign of injury to his head, such as a bruise or cut, but his right ankle was swollen and painful. David and the first responder were able to use David's mobile phone to contact his father, who said that he would meet them at the hospital. David's father spoke with his son over the phone to reassure him and then conveyed to the first responder that David didn't sound like himself to him, he sounded 'sleepy'.

Older adults

People with a learning disability tend to experience frailty associated with ageing at an earlier age than other people. Those aged 50 years and over, therefore, are considered older adults.[19] People with a learning disability may require additional support and considerations as they age, including, for example, exercises to strengthen and maintain balance, as well as assessments for risk of falls and bone health. People with a learning disability aged 50 years and older should also have equitable access to health services for older adults (such as fall clinics) at a younger age.

Talking about death and dying

People with a learning disability and autistic people with substantial support needs may be excluded from conversations and rituals (for example, going to a funeral) around death and dying. However, it is actually very important to talk openly about death and dying with individuals with a learning disability and autistic people. Advanced care plans (ACPs) are extremely useful to plan their future care, support and treatment when, for example, they are diagnosed with a terminal illness. An ACP is a person-centred process of communication, which facilitates a person's understanding, reflection and discussion of goals, values and preferences for their future care.[20] ACPs may include, for example, bucket lists, religious rituals (for example, funeral or cremation) and treatment and care options (such as pain relief and whether or not to remain at home or move into a hospice).

> **REFLECTION: Be aware and recognise symptoms**
>
> Being able to recognise symptoms associated with common health ailments has potential to make a difference to the health and wellbeing of someone you are supporting. Test your awareness by listing the symptoms that you associate with the following health conditions:
>
> - Constipation
> - Urinary tract infection
> - Irritable bowel syndrome
> - Migraine
> - Gastric reflux
>
> Once you have noted your lists, check your awareness by conducting web searches of symptoms associated with each condition.

Mental health and wellbeing

It is paramount, when supporting individuals with a learning disability and autistic individuals, to promote and maintain their mental health and wellbeing. Factors associated with promoting mental health and wellbeing include, for example, having meaningful relationships with others, having opportunities to develop new skills or hobbies, exercising, being able to help other people and practising mindfulness.

> **GLOSSARY**
>
> **Mental health** – 'a state of mental wellbeing that enables people to cope with the stresses of life, realise their abilities, learn well and work well, and contribute to their community'.[1]

Mental health conditions

Between 30% and 50% of people with a learning disability, and between 70% and 80% of autistic people, experience a mental health condition at some point in their lives. These rates are much higher than 25% of people in the general population.[2,3] The reasons people with a learning disability and autistic people have higher rates of mental health issues may include: living with long-term conditions; being more likely to experience negative life events (for example, abuse); internalising other people's negative attitudes towards them; loneliness, lower life satisfaction, and lack of social supports and reduced coping skills.[4]

> **EXPERT VOICE: Zahra**
>
> Omar's mental health is fragile, and it took me a long time to understand that. The anxiety and frustration he feels are so deep, and I just want him to feel safe. I wish more people realised that people with autism need just as much mental care as anyone else, if not more.

The seven most commonly diagnosed mental health conditions reported for autistic people are (most common first):[3]

1. Anxiety
2. Sleeping problems
3. Disruptive/impulse-control/conduct disorders (related to not being able to control urges or impulses, for example, outbursts of anger or frustration)
4. Depression
5. Obsessive compulsive disorder
6. Bipolar disorder
7. Schizophrenia.

Six diagnosed mental health conditions reported for people with a learning disability are (most common first):[5]

1. Mood disorders (including depression and bipolar disorder)
2. Anxiety
3. Schizophrenia
4. Unspecified (no specific diagnosis)
5. Personality disorder
6. Psychosis.

In addition, people with Down syndrome aged 40 years and over are at high risk of developing Alzheimer's disease (which is the most common type of dementia). This is because people with Down syndrome are born with an extra copy of chromosome 21, which causes a build up of protein in the brain, leading to dementia.[6]

Diagnosis and treatment

It can be difficult to diagnose mental health conditions in people with a learning disability and autistic people, particularly in those who require support to recognise and communicate their thoughts, emotions, moods and other possible symptoms (for example, hearing voices):

- Mental health conditions may present differently in individuals with a learning disability and autistic individuals (for example, staring into space or to the side when experiencing hallucinations).

- Diagnostic overshadowing may be an issue (see Chapter 6: Physical health and wellbeing).
- Conversely, some people's experiences of having a learning disability or being autistic overlap with symptoms of mental health problems (such as feeling overwhelmed in busy, noisy environments or finding repetitive routines and activities comforting), which can lead to misdiagnosis. For example, a high proportion of autistic people also meet the diagnostic criteria for having attention deficit hyperactivity disorder (ADHD), which means the person may experience being unable to concentrate or focus, hyperactivity or impulsiveness.[7]
- Autistic individuals can also mask their symptoms of mental health issues.

It is important to rule out possible physical reasons for the person's symptoms. For example, sudden confusion caused by a urinary tract infection.

It is vital that mental health support and treatment for individuals with a learning disability and autistic individuals are both person centred and holistic. Mental health treatments for people with a learning disability and autistic people include medication, talking therapies (such as cognitive behavioural therapy (CBT), psychodynamic or family therapy), counselling, mindfulness and relaxation exercises (such as breathing exercises).[8]

Promoting mental health and wellbeing

There are a number of ways in which you can support a person with a learning disability or an autistic person to promote their mental health and wellbeing. These include the following:

- Ensure that they live in a sensory-friendly environment.
- Create meaningful structure in the person's day, so they are not spending long periods with nothing to do, and respect their personal routines.
- Promote a healthy lifestyle (for example, diet, sleep and exercise), and provide as many opportunities as possible for the person to exercise. From supporting the person to do housework or gardening, or going for a walk in the fresh air, to dancing at home, an event or a class.
- Provide opportunities for the person to relax (for example, listening to music, reading or meeting friends).
- Provide opportunities for the person to have new experiences and develop new skills. Start small if it helps (for example, supporting the person to prepare a meal from a recipe they haven't tried before, before trying similar dishes at a new restaurant).
- Embrace the person's interests and hobbies (even if the person is autistic and their interests are very focused). Interests and hobbies

promote self-expression, making choices, self-determination and self-esteem, as well as fostering meaningful conversations and social relationships.

- Ensure effective augmented and alternative communication strategies with the person to promote receptive and expressive communication about their mental health and wellbeing.
- Support the person to understand what moods, behaviours and activities are normal for them, so that they and their supporters will recognise when they are not feeling like themselves.
- Promote self-regulation techniques, such as breathing, mindfulness or grounding exercises.
- Encourage and support the person to make reciprocal social connections with other people.
- Balance the person's support needs with their independence; this means not doing things for the person that they can do themselves.
- Promote self-advocacy as much as possible, and advocate on the person's behalf as necessary.

Self-soothe boxes

A self-soothe box is a box or container, which an individual with a learning disability or an autistic individual places personal items in that they find help to calm (soothe) them when they are feeling stressed or anxious. For example, Abena has a learning disability and she has the following items in her self-soothe box to calm her when she is feeling stressed: holiday photographs because they are happy memories; an MP3 player with a playlist of her favourite songs; hand cream with a fragrance she loves; nail polish; and a soft toy she likes to cuddle. Terence is autistic and he has the following items in his self-soothe box to calm him when he is feeling anxious: pictures of dogs because he loves dogs; a journal and pen to write down his feelings; peanut snacks; a bottle of water (for when his mouth feels dry); sound reducing headphones; fidget toys; and a silk scarf because he likes the feel of the fabric when he touches it.

Suicide safety plans

Autistic people are at much higher risk of thinking about or attempting suicide compared to other people who are not autistic. Reasons for this can include finding it challenging living in a world that is geared towards neurotypical people, mental health issues (such as depression), or being teased or bullied. Autistic individuals may also find it difficult to dispel initial thoughts about suicide because of a tendency to perseverate (which means repeated or prolonged thinking about the same thing).

A suicide safety plan is important for supporting an autistic person to recognise when they are having suicidal thoughts, feelings or urges, and for identifying the steps they can take to prevent acting on these thoughts/feelings/urges. A suicide safety plan for autistic individuals involves the individual being supported to complete relevant information about themselves, to develop coping and support strategies. This information includes: recording what is important to them (to think about things worth living for); warning signs that they may be having thoughts, feelings or urges to end their life (such as eating or sleeping less); what they can do to distract themselves (for example, breathing exercises or physical exercise); who they can contact to ask for help, particularly during a crisis; what they can do to make the environment around them safe (for example, throwing away items they can harm themselves with); and what other people need to know to help them (for example, how they communicate distress).[9]

Masking

Masking (or camouflaging) is a term used to describe autistic people hiding or disguising aspects of their self to fit in with societal norms, and behaving more in the ways neurotypical people behave in social situations. For example, mimicking other people's expressions that don't come naturally to them, forcing eye contact even though they find it uncomfortable, suppressing behaviours that usually calm them (such as hand flapping or rocking their body), not talking about intense interests they have in case other people find them odd, and trying not to flinch when another person touches them. Masking is both conscious and unconscious, and impacts negatively on the person's self-esteem, because it is associated with stigma and the person internalising negative attitudes of others about autism.[10] Masking may be protective in the sense that it enables the person to, for example, maintain relationships, feel less anxious about social situations and avoid bullying or harassment.

Masking is exhausting for an autistic person, and it is harmful to their mental health and wellbeing. Autistic people who mask are more likely to experience anxiety and depression, and may be more likely to think about or attempt suicide.[10] While society has developed an increased awareness about autism in general, there is still a lack of awareness of what it is actually like for individuals being autistic. The only way forward is to increase this awareness (to understand things from an autistic person's perspective and experience), so that autistic people know that they can be their true selves across all social situations and not have to worry about other people viewing them as different.[10]

> **REFLECTION: Talking about mental health**
>
> This exercise encourages you to practise thinking and talking about mental health and wellbeing.
>
> 1. Spend a few minutes thinking about a time recently when you were feeling stressed, low in mood or

anxious. What was the cause of this? How did being stressed, low in mood or anxious affect you? (For example, feeling irritable or angry, restless, shaking or sweating, headache, loss of appetite or sleep). What helped to make you feel better? (For example, walking in nature, phoning a friend, spending less time on social media comparing yourself to others, meditation or having a long bath).

2. Thinking about a self-soothe box, list 8–10 items that you would place in your own box. What is it about each item that is important to you and how does it help calm you?

3. Repeat steps 1 and 2 with a friend, relative or colleague. Ask them about their recent experience of stress, low mood or feeling anxious (cause, symptoms and coping strategy), as well as their choice of personal self-soothe box items.

4. If you were to repeat steps 1 and 2 with a person with a learning disability or an autistic person how would you go about it? How would you adapt your communication, and are there any accessible resources or objects of reference you would source to support receptive and expressive communication with the person? How would you use the information discussed to support the person during future instances of stress/low mood/anxiety?

Did you find it easy and insightful to talk about mental health?

Between 5% and 15% of people with a learning disability, and around 40% of autistic people, develop behaviours that challenge.[1,2] These behaviours are mainly verbal or physical aggression (for example, screaming or hitting out) or self-injury (slapping or hitting themselves), but can also refer to destructiveness to property (breaking things), sexually inappropriate behaviour, eating inedible objects and elopement (wandering from a safe environment without telling anyone). When a person displays behaviour that challenges, this does not mean that the person is challenging, but rather their behaviour is a challenge for the people who are supporting them. It would be wrong to view the person negatively as a result of their behaviour. Moreover, the person's behaviour may only occur in certain situations, and the same behaviour may only be considered challenging in some settings and circumstances but not others.[2]

GLOSSARY

Behaviours that challenge – 'Behaviour can be described as challenging when it is of such an intensity, frequency or duration as to threaten the quality

> of life and/or the physical safety of the individual or others, and it is likely to lead to responses that are restrictive, aversive or result in exclusion'.[3]

People with a learning disability are more likely to develop behaviours that challenge if they have any of the following:[2]

- A severe learning disability
- Autism
- Communication needs
- A visual impairment
- Physical health conditions
- The person is a young adult (in their teens or twenties).

People with specific genetic learning disability conditions can also be more likely to develop particular behaviours that challenge. For example, people with Lesch-Nyhan syndrome are more likely to self-harm because of a lack of dopamine ability to regulate behaviour, and people with Prader-Willi syndrome are more likely to have pica, which means eating non-food substances due to having a constant craving for food.[4] When you are supporting someone with a specific learning disability condition, it is helpful to research the condition to gain awareness and under-standing of any typical characteristics that may affect behaviour.

Causes of behaviour

All behaviour has a function, which means there is always a reason for the way the person is acting. It is important to consider a number of possible reasons for the person's behaviour. These include:[5]

- Communication needs
- Sensory needs
- Changes in the person's routine or environment
- Physical pain or discomfort (for example, toothache or ear infection)
- Physical health condition (for example, constipation or epilepsy)
- An unmet need (for example, hunger or thirst)
- Stress
- Mental health issues (for example, anxiety or depression)
- Past trauma
- Abuse
- Having little or no choice or control
- Having little or nothing to do
- Trying to avoid or escape from a situation.

EXPERT VOICE: Zahra

When Omar acts out, it's not because he is trying to be difficult; it's because he's overwhelmed, scared or unable to express himself. As a mother, all I've ever

> wanted is for people to understand his behaviour and treat it with compassion. Positive approaches have helped us to find peace in moments of chaos.

Behaviour and communication

People with a learning disability and autistic people can be more likely to exhibit behaviour that challenges if they are finding it difficult to understand what another person is saying to them or asking them to do, or if they are finding it hard to express what they want or how they are feeling.[6] This may be because of misinterpretation or feeling anxious, fearful, distressed or frustrated. It is important to understand that being an effective communication partner is key to supporting people and reduces the likelihood of behaviours that challenge. The following scenario demonstrates this.

Julie is Fred's support worker. Julie tells Fred that they will be going on his favourite walk in about 30 minutes, so not to put his jacket on yet. Fred goes to fetch his jacket but Julie stops him, saying 'No. Wait'. A few minutes later Fred starts screaming and biting his hands. Julie decides she will have to cancel their walk because of his behaviour. She doesn't realise that Fred only understood the words 'walk', 'jacket', and 'no'.

In order to be an effective communication partner, Julie needs to adapt her communication with Fred to ensure and check his understanding. The use of a pictorial activity timetable each day could help him understand what is happening and when. An alarm clock or timer could also be used to help him develop his understanding of waiting. If he is unable to wait, Julie should only mention his jacket when it is time to go for a walk. It is also important to realise that – as long as it is safe for them both to do so – still going for the walk is more likely to calm Fred than to escalate his behaviour further. Fred was not behaving badly to make Julie take him for a walk. He was upset because he thought they weren't going for a walk at all, and he feels even worse when not going for a walk is realised.

A behaviour diary

A behaviour diary is a way of recording and making sense of a person's behaviour and can help you to understand and support them in positive ways, avoid the person behaving in this way in the future, and help them to learn how to make themselves understood or have their needs met. An ABC chart – completed with support from a trained professional, such as a psychologist – is useful for capturing information about the person's behaviour.[5] Table 8.1 provides an example of how to use an ABC chart.

Table 8.1: An ABC chart example

Antecedent	Behaviour	Consequence
What happened before the behaviour? Were there any triggers? What was the context/ environment like?	What was the behaviour of concern? Be as specific and detailed as possible. For example, instead of writing 'John was hurting someone', write 'John got up from his chair, walked over to Sally and pulled her hair with both hands'.	What happened as a result of the behaviour? What was the person getting or not getting from their actions, and were there consequences that would make them want to repeat the behaviour? For example, Sally left the room.
Jake's sister Carol ran into the kitchen, where he was having breakfast, and shouted at their mother, 'Where is my schoolbag?'.	Jake thumped the table with both of his fists, knocking over a jug of orange juice.	Carol laughed and their mother shouted about the mess.

Antecedent	Behaviour	Consequence
The radio was playing loudly and the toast was burning in the toaster, setting off the smoke alarm.	When orange juice soaked the clothes he was wearing, he started crying and slapping his face.	Jake ran in to the garden and jumped on the trampoline.

Once you have charted the person's behaviour, it becomes easier to identify antecedents (or triggers) to avoid in the future, understand what the person is telling you through their actions (so you can find ways of replacing their actions with healthier and safer responses) and to reflect on consequences. In this scenario, Jake's triggers were his sister shouting, the loud radio, the smell of toast burning, the sound of the smoke alarm, unexpected disruption to his morning routine, as well as being soaked with juice. The behaviours of concern were thumping the table with his fists and slapping his face. On reflection, his sister laughing and his mother shouting made him feel worse. More positive steps to support Jake could include:

- Supporting Carol to get her schoolbag ready the evening before and leave it in the same place (for example, beside the door) so she knows where it is each morning.

- Having the radio turned off or at a low volume during breakfast.
- Ensuring the setting on the toaster will not burn the toast.
- Telling Jake it is okay about the spilt juice and helping him to clean up and change his clothes.
- Reassuring Jake that the rest of his day and routines will be as normal.
- Not laughing or shouting.
- Jake already knows that jumping on his trampoline calms him. Ask Jake if he would like to jump on his trampoline before school every morning.

Functional assessment and positive behaviour support plan

The next steps after keeping a behaviour diary are for the behavioural specialist (for example, psychologist) to conduct a functional assessment with the person and then use the information to develop a person-centred and holistic positive behaviour support (PBS) plan with them and their supporters. The purpose of a functional assessment is to understand the reason for the person's behaviour, so they can then be supported to develop other ways of getting their needs met. A PBS plan is based on a shared understanding (between the person, their supporters, and any professionals involved) of how to support the person, to reduce their behaviour that challenges and/or lessen the impact of their behaviour on themselves and those around them. A PBS plan may include, for example, supporting the person to express their feelings and needs using picture cards, supporting the person to understand and be able to cope with having to wait, and encouraging the person to be more involved in day-to-day life, such as household chores.[5]

Forensic services

There are specialist community-based forensic services throughout the UK for people with a learning disability and autistic people who have offending behaviours (for example, arson, physical aggression or sexual offences).[7] These services support individuals to access interventions and co-produce support plans.

Physical and chemical restraints

The response to individuals with a learning disability and autistic people who have behaviours that challenge must involve the least restriction necessary. Restrictive practices, such as physically restraining the person (for example, holding them down) or injecting them with a drug to calm them, should be used as a last resort and only if absolutely necessary. When these restrictions do occur they must be recorded, reported within the organisation and reviewed to guard against improper use or overuse.[8]

Autism meltdown

Autistic individuals can experience meltdowns. A meltdown is not a behaviour that challenges, but rather an involuntary loss of behaviour. It is an intense response to a situation that the person finds over-whelming, which may be characterised by the person shouting, screaming, crying, kicking or lashing out, for example. Every person is different but common causes of meltdowns can include sensory overload, a change in the person's routine when their routines are very important to them, communication issues or feeling very anxious in a situation. For example, Bartek is in a hospital's emergency department, and he cannot cope with the loud noises, bright lights and having to sit in the crowded waiting area.[9]

When a person is experiencing a meltdown, it is important to give them as much space and time as they need to recover. Do what you can to reduce the sensory overload (for example, adjust the lights and sounds, and ask other people to move along and not stare at them). Speak to the person calmly and do not place any demands on them (such as asking questions) as they recover.[9]

Marek and his support worker James are involved in a road traffic accident. Marek runs from the car, which is now stationery, but James is unable to follow him because he has sustained a whiplash injury. When Karen, who is a paramedic, arrives at the scene, two police officers are trying to prevent Marek from running into the path of oncoming traffic. Marek is extremely distressed, screaming and lashing out at the police officers.

Karen has a brother who is autistic, so she recognises that Marek may be experiencing a meltdown. She realises that she will have to approach the situation differently with Marek from how she would with someone who is not autistic. In an emergency she would usually act quickly to assess and treat the person, but she knows it is important to give Marek as much time and space as he needs first. Touching him on the arm or shoulder to comfort and reassure him, and ask questions to gather information about him and any potential injuries he may have, could worsen the distress he is experiencing. Instead, she leads him gently by the hand away from the scene and the gathering crowd, to a quiet embankment at the side of the road. She sits beside him, and tells him she is there to help.

After some time, Marek becomes aware of blood on his sweatshirt from a cut on his forehead, and he removes his sweatshirt. Karen takes this as a sign of Marek becoming calm enough to be aware of his surroundings and his bloody clothing. She asks her colleague to bring a blanket for Marek to cover himself. She helps him wrap the blanket tightly around himself, as she thinks he will find the snug feeling comforting. Once Marek is ready, and she has explained to him what will happen next and in what order, they go into the back of the ambulance. When she begins her assessment of Marek, she conducts tests from distal (away from the centre of the body) first, before proximal tests (nearer the centre of the body), in a way that he is comfortable with to reduce the likelihood of him becoming more distressed or anxious.[10]

Stimming

Stimming is common amongst autistic people, as well as some people with a learning disability. Stimming is self-stimulatory (or self-soothing) behaviour, characterised by repetitive movements, actions or sounds, which the person finds helps them cope with stressful situations.[11,12] Stimming can include, for example, hand-flapping, finger-flicking, flicking a rubber band, jumping, body-rocking, twirling a piece of string, repeating the same words or phrases, or humming. There are a number of reasons why an individual may stim. These include the person experiencing too much sensory information (for example, as a way of coping in a busy, brightly lit and noisy environment), too little sensory stimulation, to stop or lessen pain and to manage strong emotions (for example, feeling very happy or very sad).[13] It is important to understand reasons for the person's stimming, to make adaptations to their sensory environment as necessary, or support them if they are experiencing pain or feeling sad.

Autistic people who stim do report that they find this behaviour enjoyable.[12] Stimming is also beneficial for the person's mental health and wellbeing, as it is a coping mechanism that enables the person to self-regulate and manage their emotions.[13] Stimming only develops into a behaviour that challenges if it is of such frequency and intensity that it is causing harm or pain to the person or others. For example, Aki flaps her hands so often and vigorously that her hands have become swollen and red. Aki's parents are supporting her to replace her stimming behaviour with using stress balls instead.

Stimming can be misunderstood by other people because of a lack of awareness and understanding of what it is like for the person being autistic. If you are supporting someone who stims in public or social settings, it is worth taking the opportunity to raise awareness, with the person's consent and if it is appropriate, by explaining their behaviour and how it helps them. For example, explaining to another passenger on a bus that Dan is flapping his hands because he is really excited about visiting a friend at their house to meet their new puppy. He is trying to contain his excitement.

> **REFLECTION: Respond don't react**
>
> How you respond to a person influences their behaviour and the risk of their behaviour escalating. It is important to respond rather than react. A response is a well thought out action that leads to a positive outcome, whereas a reaction is fuelled by emotions, often negative. Respond to the person calmly, give them space and reassure them.
>
> Spend a few minutes thinking about a time you **reacted** negatively to another person's behaviour. What was the person's behaviour? What was causing their behaviour? How did you react? What were your thoughts and feelings that made you react this way? How would you respond differently to a similar situation?
>
> Now think about a time you **responded** positively to another person's behaviour. What was the person's behaviour? What was causing their behaviour? How did you respond? What were your thoughts and feelings that made you react this way? How did your response influence the outcome?
>
> These personal reflections will help you to understand what doesn't work and what works well when you are supporting someone who is feeling anxious, fearful, frustrated, angry or upset.

CHAPTER 9

Reasonable adjustments

People with a learning disability and autistic people access the same healthcare services as everyone else, with specialist input from, for example, community-based learning disability teams (CLDT) as appropriate. CLDTs comprise multi-disciplinary specialists in learning disability, who also provide support to people with a learning disability who are autistic.

Despite the high rates of physical and mental health issues among people with a learning disability and autistic people, they can experience barriers to accessing the same healthcare as everyone else. These barriers include a lack of AAC communication, physical barriers (such as the absence of ramps, elevators or accessible toilets) and a lack of awareness of their particular health and support needs. It is pivotal that everyone working in health services has awareness training so as to be aware of the health, communication and support needs of people with a learning disability and autistic people, in accordance with their healthcare roles.[1]

The Equality Act 2010 addresses barriers experienced by people with a disability, as it is a statutory requirement that service providers throughout the

UK make 'reasonable adjustments' to ensure people with a disability have the same equity of access to their services as everyone else.[2] We are considering reasonable adjustments in the context of health services in this chapter, but the Equality Act (2010) applies to all services throughout the UK, including employers of individuals with disabilities.

GLOSSARY

Reasonable adjustments – removing barriers and, importantly, making whatever alterations are necessary to ensure services work equally well for people with disabilities as they do for people without disabilities (United Kingdom Government, 2010).[2]

Reasonable adjustments are wide-ranging practical and affordable adjustments (there is no exhaustive list), which are often specific to a person's individual needs. For example, Marjory is autistic. She has been attending the same health centre for years but has always refused blood tests and vaccinations because she is scared of needles. A new nurse at the health centre considered reasonable adjustments with Marjory, and found that she is fine having an injection as long as a topical anaesthetic cream is applied to her arm first to reduce pain sensitivity. The nurse also found that Marjory is able to tolerate an arm cuff inflating during blood pressure monitoring if she uses a manual rather than a digital blood pressure monitor (a manual monitor does not inflate the arm cuff as quickly or as tightly as a digital one). These reasonable adjustments transform health and wellbeing. Marjory is now able to visit relatives abroad with her family, as well as have a flu vaccination in winter, and she has commenced medication to control her high blood pressure.

EXPERT VOICE: Marion

When we arrive for a hospital appointment, it would be great if the first nurse, or the first person who meets us, asks if there's anything that can be done to make things easier for Laura during the appointment.

What is reasonable?

People with a learning disability are at a higher risk of developing osteoporosis (weaker, more fragile bones), which can lead to bone fractures, so it is important that people with a learning disability are able to access bone health screening to check for and diagnose osteopenia or osteoporosis. A city-centre hospital has a DEXA (dual x-ray absorptiometry) scanner (an x-ray machine that the person lies on for their bones to be scanned), but this particular scanner is not compatible with a hoist. A hoist is a mechanical device that is used to transfer a person with a physical disability from one place to another (for example, from a wheelchair to a shower seat, bed or, in this instance, a DEXA scanner). Instead, patients who require a hoist to transfer on to a DEXA scanner are redirected to another hospital in the city, where the scanner is compatible with a hoist. This alternative arrangement is a reasonable adjustment. Excluding someone from having a scan because they use a wheelchair would not only be unreasonable but against anti-discriminatory law.

Supporting health appointments

EXPERT VOICE: Sam

When the doctor did my learning disability and autism assessment, the other people in the room were my parents, and I wasn't in the room. I had no idea about what was happening or being discussed. The doctor probably thought, because of my disability, I wouldn't engage a lot or understand him much. He probably thought I wouldn't talk to him, or understand what was going on, so he put me out of the room.

It is important to ensure health appointments for people with a learning disability and autistic people go as smoothly as possible; negative experiences can lead to them becoming anxious, worried or stressed about future appointments. When you are supporting someone, it is beneficial to notify the practice, clinic or hospital beforehand that the person has a learning disability and/or is autistic and to specify their individual reasonable adjustment needs (for example, providing a disabled car parking space or a longer appointment). Also think about how you can support the person to prepare for their appointment. For example:

- Providing accessible information about what will happen during the person's health appointment (such as an online video of someone having the same medical examination or procedure).
- Supporting the person to talk about their upcoming appointment (for example, worries or fears, symptoms, expectations and questions they will want to ask during the appointment).
- Ensuring the person has sunglasses (light sensitivity) or sound reducing headphones (noise sensitivity) or a face mask or scarf scented with a fragrance they like if they find clinical smells difficult.
- Providing things the person likes and which help them relax while waiting for their appointment (such as a fidget toy, snacks and drinks, magazines or an MP3 player with a favourite playlist).
- Ensuring the person is prepared for their appointment on the day (for example, having the

appointment scheduled on their visual timetable, and pre-booking a taxi or knowing what public transport to take and when).

EXPERT VOICE: Vicky

I would tell health professionals to offer help to learning disabled people, and just be happy and kind. I go to the doctors with my carer. They don't mind. They tell me to bring my carer in with me.

Champions and liaison nurses

Many hospitals throughout the UK have a learning disability, autism or neurodiversity champion or a liaison nurse. This is a designated person you may contact, who is responsible for liaising with clinic or ward staff to ensure the person's health, communication and support needs are met while they are at the hospital.

Reasonable adjustments in healthcare

This section provides a list of examples of reasonable adjustments that a person with a learning disability or an autistic person may require for a health appointment.[3,4,5] These examples are described in Table 9.1.

Table 9.1: Reasonable adjustment examples

Aspects of health appointment	Description and examples
Inclusive communication and augmentative and alternative communication (ACC)	Ensure all staff have good understanding of AAC and are confident communicating with individuals with a learning disability and autistic individuals.
Accessible information	Ensure all information is accessible (using easier words, pictures and symbols), from information provided on the service's website to appointment cards/letters. This also applies to having accessible signage throughout the service (such as toilet signs).
Flexible appointments	Ensure the booking system is accessible, whereby people can book appointments by telephone, online or face to face (this includes being able to amend bookings in the same way). Provide telephone reminders of upcoming appointments if that helps the person to remember and prepare for their appointment.

(Continued)

Table 9.1:   (Continued)

Aspects of health appointment	Description and examples
	Offer longer appointments (for example, double appointments) if the person needs more time for communication around symptoms, treatment and advice.
	Be flexible when arranging appointments. For example, it takes Joe's parents three hours to support him to shower, dress and eat breakfast every morning. Joe and his parents prefer appointments after 11am that do not rush or interfere with his morning routine.
	During a lengthy consultation or procedure, provide comfort breaks. Or conduct the consultation/procedure over multiple appointments.
	Allow the person to have snacks, drinks, their favourite music played or anything else that helps to relax them during the consultation or procedure.

Aspects of health appointment	Description and examples
Waiting area	If the person finds it difficult to wait in busy waiting areas, then offer appointments at less busy times (such as first or last appointment of the day). Or provide a quieter space for them away from the main waiting area.
Familiarity	Be aware that the person may prefer to see the same staff member as before, if possible, during multiple appointments. Offer familiarisation visits if it helps a person to become familiar with medical equipment or a hospital ward prior to a procedure.
Supporters	Be aware that the person may require a relative, close friend or support worker with them during appointments.
Physical environment	Ensure the environment is clutter-free and accessible. Pay attention to the person's sensory needs with regard to lighting, noise, smells, tastes and touch.

(Continued)

Table 9.1:   (Continued)

Aspects of health appointment	Description and examples
	Where possible provide ramps (including mobile ramps), hand rails (particularly at steps and stairs), elevators, colour contrasts for people with a visual impairment, a hearing loop system for people with a hearing impairment, an accessible toilet for people with a disability, and disabled parking.
Hospital stays (for example, for surgery)	A person with a learning disability or an autistic person may require sedation for treatment that they find challenging (for example, urgent dental treatment).
	If the person does find procedures challenging, consider multiple procedures under sedation at the same time (for example, a routine blood test while having teeth extracted under sedation).
	Offer a pre-admission home visit from, for example, a champion or liaison nurse, ward staff or the person's consultant or surgeon.

Aspects of health appointment	Description and examples
	Prior to planned surgery, a person's support plan may be to offer sedation at home first, or even in the hospital car park, prior to hospital admission.
	The person may find it easier to stay in a side room in a ward. If that is not possible, provide a quieter bed in a ward or allow the person to use bed curtains.
	Before and after surgery, allow the person's supporter to be with them in the anaesthetic room and the recovery room.
	Allow the person's supporter to stay with them during hospital stays (for example, on a camp bed beside their hospital bed).

EXPERT VOICE: Zahra

Simple adjustments in everyday settings make a world of difference for Omar. Whether it's reducing noise levels or providing quiet space. It's heart breaking to think how much of the world Omar has to avoid because it's too overwhelming for him. I believe health and social care sectors can do so much more to make reasonable adjustments, ensuring that individuals like Omar don't have to be excluded, and families like ours don't have to make sacrifices alone.

Hospital passports

Many people with a learning disability and autistic people have hospital passports or personalised support plans. These personalised documents contain information about the person's health, preferred communication style and support needs. It is very important that hospital staff refer to the person's passport during appointments and hospital stays, as they contain information about what the person needs them to know and understand about them during these times.

EXPERT VOICE: Marion

For nine months we were regularly phoning the doctors because we could see that our daughter was experiencing pain. Laura is unable to tell us if she has pain or where it is coming from, but it seemed to be connected to needing to empty her bladder and emptying her bladder. It was getting worse, and we filmed these episodes of extreme pain to show to a doctor; the doctor didn't want to see the film. The doctor said it was probably bladder spasms, and he didn't want to prescribe anti-spasm drugs as the drug side-effects could be worse for Laura. He recommended massaging her tummy to relax her muscles.

Eventually we asked for a longer appointment with the doctor to insist that he refer Laura to urology. This doctor told us that he wouldn't recommend sending Laura to a urology specialist, because he thought that any investigative tests would be very uncomfortable for Laura and 'not worth it'. So I asked would he just leave Laura with undiagnosed pain, and he said, 'Yes'. I suggested to him that if his daughter was in pain, he would not leave her in pain. We made the argument for Laura going to urology, and he reluctantly agreed to refer her.

With no discomfort whatsoever, Laura had a scan at the Urology department, which showed a stone in her bladder. After removing the stone, the surgeon commented that Laura must have been suffering a lot of pain because of it.

After some months, Laura was still experiencing pain, and so she was put on a hospital waiting list for a supra-pubic catheter procedure to be done. We waited eagerly for months for this, and hoped that this would mean an end to Laura's pains. The day before this planned procedure, in the afternoon, we got a phone call from the hospital to say that Laura's operation may have to be postponed, because the

Same Day Admissions Unit didn't have a hoist. Laura needs a hoist to get out of her wheelchair on to a trolley or bed. They said that Laura would have to be admitted to a hospital ward instead, as the admissions ward did have a hoist, but at present there were no beds available. They suggested we phone the admissions ward in the morning, and if there was a bed available then, they could take Laura in and the procedure would go ahead. If there wasn't a bed available then, Laura would have to go back on the surgeon's list and wait again. I couldn't believe what I was hearing!

The next morning a bed did become available, so Laura was able to have her procedure. However, it was bad enough that there wasn't a hoist in the Same Day Admissions Unit, but in my opinion, it was far worse that a member of this caring profession thought it was okay, to tell someone that they may have to suffer in pain longer because they didn't have a hoist.

REFLECTION: Making reasonable adjustments

Laura's doctor wasn't seeing her as a person beyond her disability. He did not appreciate that her parents know her better than anyone, and that they are in the best position to recognise when she is experiencing acute pain. Laura's parents correctly identified that the pain was being caused by an issue with her bladder. When they tried to use another form of communication to show that Laura was experiencing pain – video footage – the doctor didn't look at it. In doing so, he failed to consider the issue from Laura's perspective. The doctor may have mistakenly thought that he was being 'kind' to Laura by not prescribing her drugs with potential side effects, not referring her for tests he didn't think she could cope with or manage, and advising non-invasive massage, but he was seriously failing Laura because he was not treating her pain, or the cause of her pain.

Laura's doctor should have consulted with Laura's parents, as well as colleagues in urology, about the type of investigative tests Laura would be referred for, and then consider what reasonable adjustments could be implemented to enable her to complete these tests.

Once again, the availability of a hoist has come up as an example in the chapter. This is useful for demonstrating the necessary availability of this piece of equipment across different scenarios.

While there are many valid reasons why a hospital procedure or operation may be cancelled last minute (for example, if the surgeon is not available or the patient is too unwell), cancelling because a specialist but routinely used piece of equipment is not available is not one of them. In addition, the day care ward would have known all along they didn't have a hoist, not just the day before the procedure. It is unreasonable to unnecessarily admit a patient to a ward, and only if a bed becomes available, so they can access a hoist. It would have been more reasonable for the day care ward to borrow a hoist from another ward or department and carry on with the procedure as planned. The former added stress, uncertainty and worry to Laura and her family.

Inclusive communication, person-centredness and reasonable adjustments in practice ensure timely and effective care and treatment for people with a learning disability and autistic people. It is the lack of these things that is time-consuming and problematic, leading to delays, multiple appointments before appropriate action is taken, and postponements or cancellations.

Human rights

People with a learning disability and autistic people have the same human rights as everyone else in society. These statutory rights are listed in Table 10.1.[1]

Table 10.1: Human rights of UK citizens[1]

1	Right to life (for example, the right to life-saving medical treatment or police protection when a person's life is in danger).
2	Freedom from torture and inhuman and degrading treatment (having access to basics such as food, water and shelter, and being protected from harm or abuse).
3	Freedom from slavery and forced labour (for example, not being forced to work for little or no money).
4	Right to liberty and security (for example, not being unlawfully arrested or detained).
5	Right to a fair trial (for example, being considered innocent until proven guilty and having the right to legal representation).

(Continued)

Table 10.1: *(Continued)*

6	No punishment without law (for example, a court cannot give a heavier punishment than the law allows).
7	Respect for your private and family life, home and correspondence (for example, the right not to be separated from your family, and the right to maintain contact if the family is split up; also protection from telephone-tapping or publishing your personal information without your consent).
8	Freedom of thought, belief and religion (including the right to change your beliefs at any time) (for example, the right to follow religious rituals and practices).
9	Freedom of expression (the right to express your views via, for example, artwork, articles or social media).
10	Freedom of assembly and association (for example, the right to join a trade union or peacefully protest at a rally or gathering).
11	Right to marry and start a family (according to legal minimum ages for such) (includes, for example, same-sex marriage and adoption).
12	Protection from discrimination in respect of these rights and freedoms (people cannot be discriminated against according to their age, sex, race or disability among other things).

13	Right to peaceful enjoyment of your property (includes, for example, that a landlord cannot threaten or abuse a tenant, enter the home without the tenant's permission or refuse to carry out repairs to the property).
14	Right to education (includes free and compulsory primary education and accessible secondary and higher education).
15	Right to participate in free elections (the right to vote).
16	Abolition of the death penalty (no crime in the UK is punishable by death).

There are many instances that demonstrate that the rights of some people with a learning disability and autistic people are still not being respected. Let's look at the following as examples.

DNACPR orders during the COVID-19 pandemic

A 'do not attempt cardiopulmonary resuscitation' (DNACPR) order is a document that is kept in a seriously unwell patient's hospital records to state that they are not be resuscitated if their heart and breathing stops. A DNACPR order is completed by a doctor in consultation with and in respect of the expressed wishes of the individual and their family (especially if they are unable to make this decision on their own), when the person would be unlikely to survive resuscitation, has a terminal illness, would be too frail to recover or their heart or brain would become permanently damaged as a result.[2]

During the COVID-19 pandemic, there was evidence to suggest that DNACPR orders were being placed upon some individual COVID-19 patients in hospitals because of their learning disability (with 'learning disability' or 'Down syndrome' being written on the order as a reason or one of the reasons) or autism.[3] Since then, in the UK, the NHS has updated guidelines on the use of DNACPR orders within their services, to ensure the individual rights and wishes of each patient are respected at all times. These guidelines include the statement that 'learning disability, autism or dementia are not reasons to put a DNACPR on someone's record'.[2]

Hospital detainment

Any person, including people with a learning disability and autistic people, can be detained in a mental health hospital, according to mental health legislation, if they are at serious risk of harming themselves or others because of their mental health issues. Many people with a learning disability and autistic people who are detained in a mental health hospital long term, however, are being detained because of their learning disability or autism (which are not mental health conditions):[4,5]

- Of people with a learning disability and autistic people who are being detained in hospitals, 57% are far from their family and friends.
- The average length of time they spend in hospital is five years.
- Some of these people are being treated in segregation (secluded from others) over long periods of time.
- It has been found that for 41% of these people, their needs could be met more appropriately and effectively in the community, rather than hospital.

Admission to a mental health hospital should only be considered as an assessment and treatment option for people with a learning disability and autistic people who have a co-occurring mental health issue. No person should be detained in hospital longer than they absolutely need to be.

Abuse

People with a learning disability and autistic people are more likely to experience abuse, compared to people without a learning disability or autism in the general population. Different types of abuse, and warning signs to be aware of, are described in Table 10.2.[6]

Table 10.2: Different types of abuse and warning signs

Type of abuse	Warning sign examples
Physical abuse (for example, hitting, shoving, pinching or throwing things at the person)	Changes in behaviour (for example, refusing to see people or avoiding people they usually see).
Emotional abuse (for example, belittling, isolating or controlling the person)	Changes in emotional states (for example, the person is more withdrawn, anxious, fearful or sad).
Sexual abuse (for example, inappropriate touching, or coercing the person into having non-consensual sex)	Frequent or unexplained injuries (including cuts, bruises, burns or scalds, and broken bones).
Financial abuse (for example, controlling the person's money, stealing from them or not giving them enough money to live on)	Unpaid bills or missing money. Not having an adequate supply of basic necessities at home (for example, food, toiletries and medication).
Neglect (not meeting the person's basic needs)	Sexually transmitted diseases or other genital infections. The person acting out or mimicking the abuse they are experiencing.

Type of abuse	Warning sign examples
	Poor hygiene and appearance (for example, unwashed hair or clothing, or body odour).
	The person being dehydrated or malnourished.
	Unexplained weight loss.
	Over-use of physical or chemical restraint (for example, sedation).
	Being absent or less visible than usual (for example, not answering the door or phone, or missing appointments).

Hate crime

People with a learning disability and autistic people can be four times more likely to experience disability hate crime, compared to people with other forms of disability. Disability hate crime refers to criminal acts (such as threatening behaviour, verbal or physical abuse, or online abuse) that are targeted towards another person because of their disability. In one UK survey, 78% of people with a learning disability and autistic people said that they have been a victim of a hate crime, but 48% of these people did not report it to the police.[7]

If you are supporting someone with a learning disability or an autistic person who has experienced a hate crime, it is important to take this matter seriously and support them through the reporting process as necessary.

Mate crime

People with a learning disability and autistic people can also be more likely to experience mate crime. Mate crime is a form of hate crime, whereby a person deliberately befriends a person because of their disability, mental health issue, learning disability or autism to exploit them. Warning signs that a person is a victim of mate crime may include, for example, someone moving into their home and taking over (known as 'cuckooing') and/or taking control of their life (for example, what they can do and who can visit); someone displaying controlling or punishing behaviour (for example, withholding personal care or medication); or the person being exploited for financial gain (for example, someone using their mobility car or blue badge parking permit fraudulently for their own use, or claiming carers' allowance but not actually supporting the person).[8]

Troy has started travelling on a local bus to college five days per week, but since then, his parents noticed that he is hungrier than usual when he gets home and seems to be worrying about something. Troy's parents explored the possible reasons for this with him, and Troy told them about a new friend he meets on the bus, who takes money from him to buy alcohol and tobacco, so he has no money left to buy lunch. Through discussion with his parents, Troy was assured that it was okay to tell this person he wasn't going to give him any more money. He also took his parents advice to avoid this person, and sit at the front of the bus near the driver to feel safe during his journey.

> **REFLECTION: Know your rights and the rights of people you care for or support**
>
> It is important to know your rights, and the rights of people you care for or support, as well as what being able to enjoy and exercise these rights should look like in practice. Reflecting on these discriminatory examples you have just been given, which of the 16 rights (Table 10.1) do the following issues breach?
>
> - DNACPR orders with learning disability, autism or dementia written as a reason, or one of the reasons, on the order.
> - Long-term detainment in a mental health hospital.
> - Abuse.
> - Hate crime.
> - Mate crime.

Challenge and raise awareness

When you are supporting a person with a learning disability or an autistic person, it is important to be aware of adversity they can face in exercising their rights and being treated as equal citizens. Challenge discriminatory attitudes, situations and practices. Make sure the person is living in a supportive environment, where they feel safe and respected at all times. This includes providing time and space for the person to feel comfortable communicating any concerns, anxieties or worries they may have, as well as supporting the person to understand and exercise their rights. Be aware of any potential signs of harm or neglect, and act on such appropriately and sensitively.

Increasing awareness about the lives, communication and support needs of people with a learning disability and autistic people is the most effective way to support people with these conditions and to reduce stigma, marginalisation and discrimination.[9] Once you have finished reading this book, share what you have read with your friends, family and colleagues to increase awareness more widely.

Empowerment

GLOSSARY

Empowerment – a person having authority or power to do something. The process of empowerment refers to the person becoming stronger and more confident, particularly with regard to being able to control their own life (for example, make decisions) and claiming their rights.[10]

Empowerment for people with a learning disability and autistic people, who have support needs, means:[11]

- Being involved in the design and delivery of these supports and services (we call this 'co-production').
- Getting the support that is right for them.
- Being treated as equal citizens, whereby they are able to feel confident and respected by others.
- The person's values and experiences are respected and listened to.
- Providing support that enables the person to take control over their own life.
- Being able to make their own decisions. Or making decisions in their best interests if they are unable to make some decisions on their own.
- Power being with the person and not with the professionals or services.

EXPERT VOICE: Zahra

My dream is for Omar to be independent one day, but that dream sometimes feels far away. Every small step towards independence fills me with pride, but we need a system that empowers individuals like him to live a life filled with dignity and self-worth.

When you are supporting a person with a learning disability or an autistic person, the topics we have covered in this book – inclusive communication, person-centredness and reasonable adjustments – are vital for the person's empowerment. Other important points to consider are:

- Being clear to the person that they have the power to make decisions about their own life.
- Ensuring that the person has the same opportunities and freedoms as everyone else to live their life in the community.
- Ensuring that the person is living in a safe, supportive environment, and that they feel safe.
- Supporting the person to know their rights and that they can act on them.
- Providing accessible information and advice for the person to be able to make informed decisions.
- Promoting advocacy and self-advocacy.
- Building the person's self-esteem and confidence.
- Celebrating the person as an individual and never trying to make the person be someone they are not to 'fit' into society (for example, act less autistic).

Finally, living in an inclusive society means not just being aware of people with a learning disability and autistic people, but understanding what it is truly like for an individual to have a learning disability or be autistic. Hopefully this book provides some insights into that.

EXPERT VOICE: Shimara

Empowerment means being like me because I am with powerful women, black culture. Any girl's powerful, I guess, if they put their mind to it. It depends what they want to do. Let's see, like the Queen, or being a Prime Minister, or being a doctor. Empowerment for me is when I just put my mind into what I want to achieve, meaning houses, getting a job and even doing my driving lessons. Even working to do my dream job, working with special needs kids.

Communication

The Makaton Charity at http://www.makaton.org
(Makaton signs)

Widgit Online at http://www.widgit.com (accessible
pictures and symbols used in signage, visual
timetables and communication boards)

Talking Mats at http://www.talkingmats.com (a
communication system that uses symbols and other
images)

Books Beyond Words at http://www.booksbeyondwords.
co.uk (accessible picture books designed for people with
a learning disability)

Change People at http://www.changepeople.org
(provides a guide to making information accessible)

NHS England's Accessible Information Standard (2017)
standards and guidelines at: https://www.england.nhs.uk/
about/equality/equality-hub/patient-equalities-programme/
equality-frameworks-and-information-standards/
accessibleinfo/

Further information and free downloads of picture
cards and communication boards, as part of a picture
exchange communication system are available from the
following websites:

- National Autism Resources at http://www.
  nationalautismresources.com

- Pyramid Education Consultants at https://pecs-unitedkingdom.com/pecs/
- Integrated Treatment Services at http://www.integratedtreatmentservices.co.uk/speech-therapy-approaches/picture-exchange-communication-system-pecs

Physical health

A health passport template is available via the National Autistic Society website: https://www.autism.org.uk/advice-and-guidance/topics/physical-health/my-health-passport

Researchers at Kingston University in London have developed 'Growing Older: Planning Ahead' cards with people with a learning disability to help plan their future (for example, the death of a parent or transitions in care): https://www.tuffrey-wijne.com/?page_id=860

The British Institute of Learning Disabilities (BILD) has an advanced care plan (ACP) template freely available to download: https://www.bild.org.uk/resource/my-information-and-advance-care-plan-easier-read-version/

Resuscitation Council UK has developed ReSPECT, which is an accessible Recovery Summary Plan for Emergency Care and Treatment: https://www.resus.org.uk/respect/respect-healthcare-professionals

Public Health England has developed STOMP guidance on Stopping Over Medication of People with a Learning

Disability and Autistic People: https://www.england.
nhs.uk/learning-disabilities/improving-health/
stomp-stamp/

Mental health

Newcastle University has developed a suicide
safety plan for autistic people: https://research.
ncl.ac.uk/neurodisability/leafletsandmeasures/
autismadaptedsafetyplanslink/

Reasonable adjustments

Public Health England (2019) published a guide on
'Preventing falls in people with learning disabilities:
making reasonable adjustments': https://www.gov.
uk/government/publications/preventing-falls-in-people-
with-learning-disabilities/preventing-falls-in-people-with-
learning-disabilities-making-reasonable-adjustments

Improving Health and Lives: Learning Disability
Observatory (2012–2013) published a series of guides
on making reasonable adjustments for people with a
learning disability: https://www.gov.uk/government/
collections/reasonable-adjustments-for-people-with-a-
learning-disability

These guides cover the following areas:

- Blood tests
- Cancer screening
- Constipation

- Dementia
- Dysphagia
- Eye care
- Obesity and weight management
- Oral care
- Polypharmacy
- Postural care
- Preventing falls
- Substance misuse

Empowerment

Learning Disability England have published an accessible guide about 'Do Not Resuscitate (DNR) orders: Knowing your rights and challenging decisions': https://www.learningdisabilityengland.org.uk/news/latest-news/dnar-a-guide-for-understanding-your-rights-and-challenging-decisions/

Autism Speaks have developed a downloadable road map to self-empowerment for autistic adults: https://www.autismspeaks.org/roadmap/roadmap-self-empowerment-autistic-adults

1: People with a learning disability and autistic people

1. NHS England (2023). Involving people with a learning disability, autistic people, and family carers: Making information and the words we use accessible. https://www.england.nhs.uk/learning-disabilities/about/get-involved/involving-people/making-information-and-the-words-we-use-accessible/#autism

2. World Health Organization (2022). *International Classification of Diseases and Related Health Problems* (11th edn) (ICD-11). WHO: Geneva, Switzerland.

3. World Health Organization (2007). *International Statistical Classification of Diseases and Related Health Problems*. WHO: Geneva, Switzerland.

4. Department of Health (2001). *Valuing People: A new strategy for learning disability for the 21st century*. Department of Health: London, UK.

5. Department of Health (2023). Learning disability: Applying All Our Health. https://www.gov.uk/government/publications/learning-disability-applying-all-our-health/learning-disabilities-applying-all-our-health

6. Holland, K. (2011). *Factsheet: Learning disabilities*. British Institute of Learning Disabilities. https://www.moodcafe.co.uk/media/42753/BILD%20Learning_Disabilities_11.pdf

7. American Psychiatric Association (2022). Neurodevelopmental disorders. In *Diagnostic and Statistical Manual of Mental Disorders* (5th edn). American Psychiatric Association: Washington DC, USA.

8. National Institute for Mental Health (2022). Autism spectrum disorder. https://www.nimh.nih.gov/health/publications/autism-spectrum-disorder

9. Kapp, S.K., Gillespie-Lynch, K., Sherman, L.E. et al. (2013). Deficit, difference, or both? Autism and neurodiversity. *Developmental Psychology*, 49(1): 59.

10. Pellicano, E. and den Houting, J. (2022). Annual Research Review: Shifting from 'normal science' to neurodiversity in autism science. *Journal of Child Psychology and Psychiatry*, 63(4): 381–396.

11. World Health Organization (2022). Autism. https://www.who.int/news-room/fact-sheets/detail/autism-spectrum-disorders

12. Rahman, R., Reid, C., Kloer, P. et al. (2024). A systematic review of literature examining the application of a social model of health and wellbeing. *European Journal of Public Health*, 34(3): 467–472.

13. Khan, S., Combaz, E. and McAslan Fraser, E. (2015). *Social Exclusion: Topic guide*. Governance and Social Development Resource Centre, University of Birmingham: Birmingham, UK.

2: Supporting choices and decision making

1. Mental Welfare Commission Scotland (2021). *Supported Decision Making: Good practice guide.* Mental Welfare Commission Scotland: Edinburgh, UK.
2. Harding, R. (2017). What is legal capacity? Legal Capacity Research, University of Birmingham. https://legalcapacity.org.uk/everyday-decisions/what-is-legal-capacity/
3. Northern Ireland Assembly (2016). *Mental Capacity Act (Northern Ireland) 2016.* Northern Ireland Assembly: Belfast, UK. https://www.legislation.gov.uk/nia/2016/18/contents/enacted
4. UK Government (2005). *Mental Capacity Act 2005.* UK Government: London, UK. https://www.legislation.gov.uk/ukpga/2005/9/contents
5. Scottish Government (2000). *Adults with Incapacity (Scotland) Act 2000.* Scottish Government: Edinburgh, UK. https://www.legislation.gov.uk/asp/2000/4/contents
6. Boardman, L., Bernal, J. and Hollins, S. (2014). Communicating with people with intellectual disabilities: A guide for general psychiatrists. *Advances in Psychiatric Treatment*, 20(1): 27–36.
7. Finlay, W.M.L. and Lyons, E. (2002). Acquiescence in interviews with people with mental retardation. *Mental Retardation*, 40(1): 14–29.
8. Rozenkrantz, L., D'Mello, A.M. and Gabrieli, J.D. (2021). Enhanced rationality in autism spectrum disorder. *Trends in Cognitive Sciences*, 25(8): 685–696.

9. Luke, L., Clare, I.C., Ring, H., Redley, M. and Watson, P. (2012). Decision-making difficulties experienced by adults with autism spectrum conditions. *Autism*, 16(6): 612–621.

3: Support in daily life

1. National Autistic Society (2020). Dealing with change – A guide for all audiences. National Autistic Society: London, UK.
2. The Health Foundation (2016) Person-centred care made simple: What everyone should know about person-centred care. The Health Foundation: London, UK.
3. Mansell, J., Felce, D., Jenkins, J. et al. (1983). A Wessex home from home: A staffed house for mentally handicapped adults. *Nursing Times*, 79: 51–56.
4. Mansell, J., Felce, D., Jenkins, J. et al. (1987). *Developing Staffed Housing for People with Mental Handicaps*. Costello: Tunbridge Wells, UK.
5. Mansell, J. and Beadle-Brown, J. (2012). *Active Support: Enabling and empowering people with intellectual disabilities*. Kingsley: London, UK.
6. Hume, L., Khan, N. and Reilly, M. (2024). *Enabling Capable Environments Using Practice Leadership*. Pavilion Publishing: West Sussex, UK.
7. Beadle-Brown, J., Murphy, B. and Bradshaw, J. (2017). *Person-Centred Active Support* (2nd edn). Pavilion: Hove, UK.

8. UK Government (2014). Care Act 2014. UK Government: London, UK.

9. Ward, C. (2012). *BILD Factsheet*: *Older people with a learning disability*. British Institute of Learning Disabilities: Birmingham, UK.

10. National Institute for Health and Care Excellence (2018). *Care and Support of People Growing Older with Learning Disabilities*. National Institute for Health and Care Excellence: London, UK.

11. Finlayson, J., Jackson, A., Mantry, D. et al. (2015). The provision of aids and adaptations, risk assessments, and incident reporting and recording procedures in relation to injury prevention for adults with intellectual disabilities: Cohort study. *Journal of Intellectual Disability Research*, 59(6): 519–529.

4: Inclusive communication with people with a learning disability

1. World Health Organization (2007). *International Statistical Classification of Diseases and Related Health Problems* (11th edn) (ICD-11). WHO: Geneva, Switzerland.

2. Mencap (2008). *Communicating with People with a Learning Disability*. Mencap: London, UK. file:///C:/Users/heath/AppData/Local/Temp/ MicrosoftEdgeDownloads/53a090f3-0d37-498e- b2b3-72cb39529322/Your%20guide%20to%20 communicating%20with%20people%20with%20 a%20learning%20disability.pdf

3. Salford Integrated Care Partnership (2024). Speak up Salford: Information carrying words. https://www.speakupsalford.nhs.uk/information-carrying-words

4. Royal College of Speech and Language Therapists (2023). *Augmentative and Alternative Communication (AAC)*. RCSLT: London, UK. file:///C:/Users/heath/AppData/Local/Temp/MicrosoftEdgeDownloads/3b00aac0-ede4-4c15-b466-93ff944093ab/Augmentative%20and%20alternative%20communication.pdf

5. Leicestershire Partnership NHS Trust (2019). *Children's Speech and Language Therapy Service: Objects of reference*. Leicestershire Partnership NHS Trust: Leicester. https://www.leicspart.nhs.uk/wp-content/uploads/2019/02/Objects-of-Reference.pdf

6. West, E. (2024). My autism and sign language. British Deaf News. https://www.britishdeafnews.co.uk/autism-sign-language/

7. NHS England (2017). The Accessible Information Standard. https://www.england.nhs.uk/about/equality/equality-hub/patient-equalities-programme/equality-frameworks-and-information-standards/accessibleinfo/

5: Inclusive communication with autistic people

1. Capanna-Hodge, R. (2024). Neurotypical vs neurodivergent communication: Embracing diversity

in dialogue. https://drroseann.com/neurotypical-vs-neurodivergent-communication-embracing-diversity-in-dialogue/

2. Connected Speech Pathology (2024). Understanding autism and communication difficulties in adults. https://connectedspeechpathology.com/blog/understanding-autism-and-communication-difficulties-in-adults

3. Dawes, V. (2023). *Autistic Meltdowns, Burnout and First Responders*. National Police Autism Association. https://www.autisticadvocate.co.uk/_files/ugd/14d85f_824e9f7c7ed24b2c861cb4c497f72c6e.pdf

4. Milton, D.E.M. (2012). On the ontological status of autism: The 'double empathy problem'. *Disability & Society*, 27(6): 883–887.

5. Richmond, J. and Baicher, V. (2022). Communicating with neurodivergent patients. Don't Forget the Bubbles. https://dontforgetthebubbles.com/step-it-up-communicating-with-neurodivergent-patients/

6. European Council of Autistic People & Autism Europe (2022). *Supporting Autistic People in Crisis Situations*. EUCAP. https://eucap.eu/wp-content/uploads/2022/03/autism-in-crisis-printable-EN.pdf

7. Brignell, A., Chenausky, K.V., Song, H. et al. (2018). Communication interventions for autistic spectrum disorder in minimally verbal children. *Cochrane Database Systematic Reviews*, 2018(11): CD012324.

6: **Physical health and wellbeing**

1. Cooper, S.-A. and Kogan, C.S. (2023). Disorders of intellectual development. In Tyrer, P. (ed.), *Making Sense of ICD-11 for Mental Health Professionals*. Cambridge University Press: Cambridge, UK.
2. Williams, E., Buck, D., Babalola, G. et al. (2020). What are health inequalities? The King's Fund. https://www.kingsfund.org.uk/insight-and-analysis/long-reads/what-are-health-inequalities
3. Learning Disabilities Mortality Review Programme (LeDeR) (2022). *Learning Disabilities Mortality Review (LeDeR) Annual Report, 1st April 2021 to 31st March 2022: Learning from deaths of people with a learning disability*. NHS England, University of Bristol. https://bnssghealthiertogether.org.uk/wp-content/uploads/2024/10/LeDeR_Annual_Report_2021-221.pdf
4. Office for National Statistics (2023). Deaths registered in England and Wales: 2022. https://www.ons.gov.uk/peoplepopulationandcommunity/birthsdeathsandmarriages/deaths/bulletins/deathsregistrationsummarytables/2022
5. Public Health England (2018). *Health Inequalities: Cancer*. Public Health England. file:///C:/Users/heath/AppData/Local/Temp/MicrosoftEdgeDownloads/14524410-9b5f-4f8f-a254-5ae3b7ae6a1a/Health_inequalities_cancer.pdf
6. Guan, J. and Li, G. (2017). Characteristics of unintentional drowning deaths in children with autism spectrum disorder. *Injury Epidemiology*, 4: 32.

7. Learning Disabilities Mortality Review Programme (LeDeR) (2020). *Constipation – Dying for a poo.* Learning into Action Bulletin. https://www.bristol.ac.uk/media-library/sites/sps/leder/ConstipationJANnewsletter.pdf

8. Autism Speaks (2017) Autism and health: A special report by Autism Speaks. Autism Speaks: New York, USA.

9. Ward, J.H., Weir, E., Allison, C. et al. (2023). Increased rates of chronic physical health conditions across all organ systems in autistic adolescents and adults. *Molecular Autism*, 14(1): 35.

10. Liao, P., Vajdic, C., Trollor, J. et al. (2021). Prevalence and incidence of physical health conditions in people with intellectual disability – A systematic review. *PloS One*, 16(8): pe0256294.

11. Rydzewska, E., Dunn, K. and Cooper, S.A. (2021). Umbrella systematic review of systematic reviews and meta-analyses on comorbid physical conditions in people with autism spectrum disorder. *British Journal of Psychiatry*, 218(1): 10–19.

12. Kinnear, D., Morrison, J., Allan, L. et al. (2018). Prevalence of physical health conditions and multimorbidity in a cohort of adults with intellectual disabilities with and without Down syndrome. *British Medical Journal Open*, 8(2): e018292.

13. Finlayson, J., Morrison, J., Jackson, A. et al. (2010). Injuries, falls and accidents among adults with intellectual disabilities. Prospective cohort study. *Journal of Intellectual Disability Research*, 54(11): 966–980.

14. Sun, J.J., Perera, B., Henley, W. et al. (2020). Seizure and sudden unexpected death in epilepsy (SUDEP) characteristics in an urban UK intellectual disability service. *Seizure*, 80: 18–23.
15. Center for Disease Control and Prevention (2024). Sudden unexpected death in epilepsy. https://www.cdc.gov/epilepsy/sudep/index.html
16. Ogley, R., Javaid, A. and Chear, L.J. (2024). Non-pharmacological interventions in ID patients with challenging behaviours. *Progress in Neurology and Psychiatry*, 28(2): 9–14.
17. Public Health England (2024). *Health Inequalities: Sexual health*. Public Health England. file:///C:/Users/heath/AppData/Local/Temp/MicrosoftEdgeDownloads/27da51a3-3919-4a73-bde4-efd992ad5686/Health%20Inequalities_Sexual%20health.pdf
18. Hermans, H. and Evenhuis, H.M. (2014). Multimorbidity in older adults with intellectual disabilities. *Research in Developmental Disabilities*, 35(4): 776–783.
19. Voss, H., Vogel, A., Wagemans, A.M. et al. (2017). Advance care planning in palliative care for people with intellectual disabilities: A systematic review. *Journal of Pain and Symptom Management*, 54(6): 938–960.

7: **Mental health and wellbeing**

1. World Health Organization (2022). Fact sheet: Mental health. https://www.who.int/news-room/fact-sheets/detail/mental-health-strengthening-our-response

2. Inclusion Europe (2023). Mental health of people with intellectual disabilities and family members. https://www.inclusion-europe.eu/mental-health-people-intellectual-disabilities-families/

3. Lai, M.C., Kassee, C., Besney, R. et al. (2019). Prevalence of co-occurring mental health diagnoses in the autism population: A systematic review and meta-analysis. *Lancet Psychiatry*, 6(10): 819–829.

4. National Autistic Society (2021). *Good Practice Guide: For professionals delivering talking therapies for autistic adults and children*. National Autistic Society: London, UK. https://s2.chorus-mk.thirdlight.com/file/24/asDKIN9as.kIK7easFDsalAzTC/NAS-Good-Practice-Guide-A4.pdf

5. Mazza, M.G., Rossetti, A., Crespi, G. et al. (2020). Prevalence of co-occurring psychiatric disorders in adults and adolescents with intellectual disability: A systematic review and meta-analysis. *Journal of Applied Research in Intellectual Disabilities*, 33(2): 126–138.

6. Fortea, J., Zaman, S.H., Hartley, S. et al. (2021). Alzheimer's disease associated with Down syndrome: A genetic form of dementia. *Lancet Neurology*, 20(11): 930–942.

7. Hours, C., Recasens, C. and Baleyte, J.M. (2022). ASD and ADHD comorbidity: What are we talking about? *Front Psychiatry*, 13: 837424.

8. Burke, C.K. (2014). *Feeling Down: Improving the mental health of people with learning disabilities*. Foundation for People with Learning Disabilities: London, UK. file:///C:/Users/heath/AppData/Local/Temp/MicrosoftEdgeDownloads/506cad32-ea7f-4f6c-afad-ac758f7509a5/feeling-down-report-2014.pdf

9. Rodgers, J., Goodwin, J., Nielsen, E. et al. (2023). Adapted suicide safety plans to address self-harm, suicidal ideation, and suicide behaviours in autistic adults: Protocol for a pilot randomised controlled trial. *Pilot and Feasibility Studies*, 9(1): 31.
10. Belcher, H. (2022). Autistic people and masking. National Autistic Society. https://www.autism.org.uk/advice-and-guidance/professional-practice/autistic-masking

8: **Understanding behaviour**

1. Edelson, S.M. (2022). Understanding challenging behaviors in autism spectrum disorder: A multi-component, interdisciplinary model. *Journal of Personalized Medicine*, 12(7): 1127.
2. National Institute of Health and Care Excellence (2015). *Challenging Behaviour and Learning Disabilities: Prevention and interventions for people with learning disabilities whose behaviour challenges [NG11]*. NICE. https://www.nice.org.uk/guidance/ng11/resources/challenging-behaviour-and-learning-disabilities-prevention-and-interventions-for-people-with-learning-disabilities-whose-behaviour-challenges-pdf-1837266392005
3. Royal College of Psychiatrists (2007) Challenging behaviour: A unified approach. Royal College of Psychiatrists: London, UK.
4. Waite, J., Heald, M., Wilde, L. et al. (2014). The importance of understanding the behavioural phenotypes of genetic syndromes associated with

intellectual disability. *Paediatrics and Child Health*, 24(10): 468–472.

5. The Challenging Behaviour Foundation (2022). *Finding the Reasons for Challenging Behaviour: Part 2*. The Challenging Behaviour Foundation. https://www.challengingbehaviour.org.uk/wp-content/uploads/2021/02/002-Finding-the-Reasons-for-Challenging-Behaviour-Part-2-1.pdf

6. The Challenging Behaviour Foundation (2023). *Communication and Challenging Behaviour*. The Challenging Behaviour Foundation. https://www.challengingbehaviour.org.uk/wp-content/uploads/2024/12/004-Communication-and-Challenging-Behaviour-2024.pdf

7. McKinnon, I., Whitehouse, E., Harris, M. et al. (2024). A UK-wide survey of community forensic services for adults with intellectual disability and/or autism. *British Journal of Psychology Open*, 10(5): 148.

8. National Institute of Health and Care Excellence (2015). *Learning Disability: Behaviour that challenges quality standard [QS 101]*. NICE. https://www.nice.org.uk/guidance/qs101/resources/learning-disability-behaviour-that-challenges-pdf-75545232605125

9. National Autistic Society (2024). Meltdowns – A guide for all audiences. https://www.autism.org.uk/advice-and-guidance/topics/behaviour/meltdowns/all-audiences

10. Rzucidlo, S.F. (2003). *Autism 101 for EMS Practitioners*. https://www.hscfire.com/asd/docs/autism101-ems.pdf

11. National Autistic Society (2020). Stimming – A guide for all audiences. https://www.autism.org.uk/advice-and-guidance/topics/about-autism/repeated-movements-and-behaviour-stimming

12. Kapp, S.K., Steward, R., Crane, L. et al. (2019). 'People should be allowed to do what they like': Autistic adults' views and experiences of stimming. *Autism*, 23(7): 1782–1792.

13. Mitchell, K. (2024). Stimming and autism – Are they related? WebMD UK Limited: London, UK. https://www.webmd.com/brain/autism/what-you-need-to-know-about-stimming-and-autism

9: Reasonable adjustments

1. UK Government (2022). Health and Care Act 2022. https://www.legislation.gov.uk/ukpga/2022/31/contents

2. UK Government (2010). Equality Act 2010. https://www.legislation.gov.uk/ukpga/2010/15/contents

3. Haydon, C., Doherty, M. and Davidson, I.A. (2021). Autism: Making reasonable adjustments in healthcare. *British Journal of Hospital Medicine*, 82(12): 1–11.

4. Moloney, M., Hennessy, T. and Doody, O. (2021). Reasonable adjustments for people with intellectual disability in acute care: A scoping review of the evidence. *BMJ Open*, 11(2): e039647.

5. Finlayson, J., De Amicis, L., Gallacher, S. et al. (2019). Reasonable adjustments to provide equitable and inclusive assessment, screening and

treatment of osteoporosis for adults with intellectual disabilities: A feasibility study. *Journal of Applied Research in Intellectual Disabilities*, 32(2): 300–312.

10: Empowerment

1. UK Government (1998). Human Rights Act 1998. https://www.legislation.gov.uk/ukpga/1998/42/contents
2. National Health Service (2023). Do not attempt cardiopulmonary resuscitation (DNACPR) decisions. https://www.nhs.uk/tests-and-treatments/do-not-attempt-cardiopulmonary-resuscitation-dnacpr-decisions/
3. Bows, H. and Herring, J. (2022). DNACPR decisions during Covid-19: An empirical and analytical study. *Medical Law Review*, 30(1): 60–80.
4. National Autistic Society (2024). Missed target to reduce the number of autistic people detained in mental health hospitals. https://www.autism.org.uk/what-we-do/news/missed-target-to-reduce-number-of-autistic-people
5. Hollins, S. (2021). Independent care (education) and treatment reviews: An independent report and recommendations from Baroness Hollins and the oversight panel's review of the independent care (education) and treatment reviews. Department of Health. https://www.gov.uk/government/publications/independent-care-education-and-treatment-reviews

6. Ann Craft Trust (2018). Disability and domestic abuse. https://www.anncrafttrust.org/resources/disability-domestic-abuse/
7. Dimensions UK (2017). Hate crime statistics. https://dimensions-uk.org/dimensions-campaigns/i-am-a-politician-or-journalist/hate-crime-statistics/
8. Thomas, P. (2011). 'Mate crime': Ridicule, hostility and targeted attacks against disabled people. *Disability & Society*, 26(1): 107–111.
9. National Health Service (2019). NHS long term plan. https://www.england.nhs.uk/publication/the-nhs-long-term-plan/
10. Oxford University Press (2020). *The Oxford Dictionary*. Oxford University Press: Oxford, UK.
11. NHS England (2024). Why is it important to involve people. https://www.england.nhs.uk/learning-disabilities/about/get-involved/involving-people/why-is-it-important-to-involve-people/